Advance Praise for *The God Shot*

"*The God Shot* is a rare and essential work that bridges personal courage, scientific clarity, and clinical innovation. Dr. Eugene Lipov's deeply human journey—from witnessing and surviving intergenerational trauma to discovering the application of the stellate ganglion block for the treatment of trauma—anchors this groundbreaking contribution to medicine and trauma recovery. His work reframes trauma not as a psychiatric disorder, but as a neurobiological condition characterized by altered autonomic state regulation—a functional dysregulation of the autonomic nervous system, rather than a structural injury. This reframing is powerfully aligned with the principles of Polyvagal Theory.

"By interrupting the persistent state of sympathetic arousal that characterizes traumatic stress injury, the stellate ganglion block restores access to the vagus nerve's calming and anti-inflammatory mechanisms. This shift enables the return of the body's natural capacity for homeostasis, growth, restoration, and sociality—functions that are foundational to healing and human connection.

"For those who have suffered, it offers accessible hope. Dr. Lipov's compassionate mission—to lessen the burden of suffering through scientific innovation—is not only inspiring, but urgently needed. *The God Shot* opens a new chapter in trauma care, where relief is made more available, more effective, and more humane."

—Stephen W. Porges, PhD

"*The God Shot* provides a compelling and urgent narrative that echoes the neurobiological truths we are uncovering about trauma, healing, and human connection. From the vantage point of oxytocin science, this book powerfully illustrates the potential to reframe trauma not as a life sentence but as an injury—one that, like the oxytocin system itself, is sensitive to context, capable of repair, and deeply embedded in our evolutionary biology. Eugene Lipov's engaging story and his clinical solutions resonate with the principles outlined in our basic science research. Healing is not only neurochemical but relational. Safety cues, social engagement, and autonomic recalibration are central to recovery and deeply biological and resilience can be restored when we engage the body's own biobehavioral resources for regeneration and connection."

—Sue Carter, PhD, Professor of Psychology,
University of Virginia, Charlottesville

THE
GOD SHOT

THE GOD SHOT

Healing Trauma's Legacy: THE SCIENCE, THE STORIES, THE SOLUTION

DR. EUGENE LIPOV M.D.
& LAUREN UNGELDI

Post Hill Press

A POST HILL PRESS BOOK
ISBN: 979-8-89565-295-4
ISBN (eBook): 979-8-89565-296-1

The God Shot:
Healing Trauma's Legacy: The Science, the Stories, the Solution

Cover design by Conroy Accord

This book contains advice and information relating to health care. It should be used to supplement rather than replace the advice of your doctor or another trained health professional. You are advised to consult your health professional with regard to matters related to your health, and in particular regarding matters that may require diagnosis or medical attention. While all efforts have been made to assure the accuracy of the information in this book as of the date of publication, many names and identifying details have been changed to protect the privacy of the people involved. The publisher and the author disclaim liability for any medical outcomes that may occur as a result of applying the methods suggested in this book.

Post Hill Press
New York • Nashville
posthillpress.com

Published in the United States of America
1 2 3 4 5 6 7 8 9 10

Disclaimer:

This book explores real-life experiences with trauma, including stories of loss, violence, and personal struggle. Some content may be emotionally intense or triggering for certain readers. If you encounter a section that feels overwhelming, please listen to your instincts—take a break, skip ahead, or return when you feel ready.

The intention of this book is not to dwell on pain, but to offer hope, healing, and real solutions. This book is for informational purposes only; it is not intended to diagnose, treat, or replace professional medical or psychiatric advice. Always consult with a licensed healthcare provider before making changes related to your health or mental well-being.

Take what serves you, leave what doesn't, and above all, remember:

You are not alone. Keep the hope alive.

To my wife, Robbin—for her heart, her care, her humor, and for always keeping me grounded.

To my brother—whose intelligence and medical intuition inspired me to explore the potential of the Stellate Ganglion Block beyond the bounds of conventional medicine.

And to my son—for his determination, his wit, and the way he completes our family.

ACKNOWLEDGMENTS

To Linda and Glenn Greenberg—for their incredible support in turning an idea into reality, helping to transform the mental health landscape, and empowering our team to change and save lives.

We want to recognize two amazing organizations. That's how people make a difference every day. Erase PTSD Now and PenFed, through their continuous efforts, have helped improve lives. A portion of book sales will be donated to these organizations.

CONTENTS

CHAPTER 1
ORIGIN STORY OF A TRAUMA INNOVATOR

"Who is Eugene Lipov, MD?"

If you asked a hundred people who've crossed paths with me throughout my life that question, you'd likely get a hundred different answers.

Some might call me a trauma expert, an anesthesiologist, or a pain doctor. A few might, with a smirk, refer to me as the "needle plunger"—a nickname from a few dubious colleagues, not because of any secret drug habit, but because one of the biggest breakthroughs of my career involved treating trauma with the push of a needle. Others might label me a trailblazer in trauma treatment, pushing the boundaries of what's possible in modern medicine.

There's someone out there who might even tell you that I saved their loved one from suicide.

And then, out of those hundred, at least one would laugh and call me a crazy crockpot. That's thanks to my unorthodox methods, my relentless curiosity, and my refusal to accept the status quo.

For the most part, they'd all be right—except for the fellow who called me a crockpot; I'd like to think he's wrong. But then again, maybe a touch of madness is necessary for anyone bold enough to try and change the world.

But my story didn't start with a white coat and a hospital badge. In fact, it began long before I was even born. Trauma, as we now know, has the power to flip genetic switches, altering gene expression across generations—a phenomenon called epigenetic inheritance. While this doesn't change the DNA itself, it leaves an imprint that ripples through time. This gene malleability means that the echoes of trauma don't just stop with those who experienced it firsthand. It extends to their children and grandchildren, perpetuating a cycle of inherited pain and resilience.

This means that long before I took my first breath, trauma had already shaped me. The scars of my ancestors were woven into my very DNA—a silent inheritance passed down through a lineage marred by war and suffering. Though invisible, this legacy shaped me in ways both subtle and profound. I didn't know it as a child, but that genetic imprint made me more susceptible to developing PTSD than someone born with different DNA.

So, my story begins with my grandfather, a survivor of the brutal atrocities that ravaged Ukraine in the early 1900s. My father was born in 1925, just in time to be swept into the storm of World War II. Thrust into the heart of that conflict, he joined a squadron of 10,000 young men—thousands thrown into the furnace of war, facing death at every turn. When the dust finally settled, only a hundred of those men returned home. My father was one of them.

But the scars he carried weren't merely physical; they were etched deep into his soul, shaping the man he would become and how he would raise his children. The traumatic events he endured didn't just end with him; they became a part of our family's very DNA.

My father was a war hero and a physician—a man whose brilliance was matched only by the depth of the scars he carried. While he survived the Second World War, most of his friends did not. He saw things that most cannot imagine. His temper was like a tightly coiled spring, ready to snap at any moment. Living with him was like navigating a minefield—one wrong move and the explosion of rage that followed could leave us all shattered. Our home wasn't a sanctuary—it was a battleground, where my mother, brother, and I lived on edge, constantly trying to avoid becoming casualties of his private war. His anger left emotional bruises that mirrored the physical ones he must have endured.

I was born in 1958 in Cherkasy, Ukraine, just a few hours from Kyiv. Cherkasy was more than just my hometown; it was a stronghold of resilience, a place where survival wasn't just a necessity—it was an art form. The city made history as a fierce battleground during World War II, the site of the Battle of Korsun–Cherkassy, part of a massive Soviet offensive that sought to push the German forces out of Ukraine.

This was more than just a footnote in history books; it was a living, breathing part of our heritage, etched into the streets and stories of Cherkasy, shaping the lives of everyone who called it home.

My mother, a physician like my father, was the epitome of strength and sacrifice, balancing her professional aspirations with the harsh realities of postwar life. But over time, the relentless strain of living with my father's unchecked rage began to wear her down. The vibrant woman she once was gradually faded into a shadow of her former self, her spirit eroded by the constant tension that filled our home. My father's unhealed trauma was like a virus, infecting every corner of our lives—it spread through our household, taking hold of my mother, wrapping around her until her bright eyes dimmed under the weight of unspoken fears and relentless anxiety.

She tried to be the glue that held us together, but the emotional and psychological assaults frayed her nerves and sapped her strength. The joy she once found in her work and family was slowly replaced by a weary resignation, and her smile became an increasingly rare sight—an echo of the woman she used to be.

My parents were the kind of people who, in another place and time, might have lived comfortably in a plush home on a quiet corner block. But this was Cherkasy, where work was as scarce as warmth in winter. We lived in a small, two-bedroom house, where the bare walls only seemed to amplify the emptiness within. The furniture was purely functional, reflecting a life defined by frugality and simplicity, with no room for luxuries. There were no pictures on the walls, no trinkets or ornaments to add a personal touch. My parents shared one room, my brother and I slept in the living room. Every morning, I packed away my bedding to make room for the day's activities. Our home was a stark reflection of our reality: survival was our primary concern, and comfort was a luxury we couldn't afford.

There is very little that I remember clearly about my childhood; in fact, the vast mental archives where most people file and store thousands of young memories are largely empty for me. The brain has a way of protecting itself, and mine, faced with the burden of storing dozens of traumatic memories, decided it was better to wipe the old disk clean than to play a hundred recordings of my father's rage, my mother's screams, and the stinging pain on my backside from repeated beatings. But there are a few memories that somehow survived the sweep.

I remember the cold—those frigid, bleak, gray winters when the chill didn't just stay outside, it seeped into every corner of our house and every inch of my skin. No amount of layers could keep it at bay. As a child, I didn't even realize how poor we were until the winter I turned six, when our home became an icebox. I asked my mother why she'd stopped adding coal to the stove, and her answer was simple: We didn't have money to buy any. The cold wasn't just a temperature; it was a presence, creeping into our bones and settling deep within.

Beyond the cold, I remember my mother making herring and mashed potatoes with garlic. She hated cooking and wasn't particularly good at it, but—somehow—the mashed potatoes and herring always turned out well. It was our little culinary miracle amidst the bleakness, a small comfort in a world that offered so few.

Family vacations to Sochi, along the Black Sea in Southern Russia, were nothing short of torture, and I hated them with a passion. It wasn't just the fact that the Black Sea was rumored to be 70 percent urine from all the vacationers, it was the fact that without the distractions of daily life, we bore the full brunt of my father's tumultuous moods. My mother and I would try to maintain a fragile peace, walking a tightrope that often ended with us being the next targets. I lived in perpetual fear that

I would say or do the wrong thing and provoke him to violence. There was no pattern or predictability to his outbursts—if there had been, I would have tried to crack the code to avoid the inevitable pain. My father wasn't a monster, though he certainly seemed like one at times. He was brilliant and thoughtful, but he was a war hero who could never seem to win the battle raging in his own mind. My mother and I just happened to get caught in the crossfire.

Aside from the bitter cold of those bleak Ukrainian winters, the garlic mashed potatoes and herring, and the sound of my father's shouts on family vacations, there is only one other memory that stands out from the summer when I was six years old.

I gathered with a small group of neighborhood boys I liked to play with when the weather was nice. That day, we stumbled upon a big, rusty-looking pipe.

"What is it?" one of the boys, several years older than me, asked, tapping it with his toes.

No one knew, but one of the boys stooped down and picked it up. It was heavy, but he carried that old thing back with us, triumphant.

"Look what we found!" I exclaimed to my father when we showed him. My father took one look at the rusty old pipe in my friend's hands and lurched forward, snatching it away faster than a whip—steady and calculated.

"Don't EVER play with this or touch it again!" my father yelled. He was a seasoned veteran, and he knew enough to recognize an unexploded artillery shell when he saw one.

Later that day, my father walked carefully with it into a forest that bordered our little town and buried it deep in the earth. The next day, my friends were back with that same gleam in their eyes.

"Want to come and play with us?" they asked, innocently enough, when I answered the door.

"Absolutely not," my father said before I had time to reply.

I was furious, but my father was insistent. I knew better than to sulk; my father hated it with a passion, and I didn't want to make him angrier. I tried to keep myself busy, but inside, I was having one big pity party. Then we heard the explosion.

We later learned that the boys had discovered where my father buried the artillery shell and dug it up. Overcome by curiosity, they hit it against a tree. When nothing happened, they decided to throw a rock at it. And then something *did* happen.

One boy lost an arm and a leg; the other lost both legs. At six years old, my two best friends were blown up and mangled, and I was never the same. From that day on, I began to plan an escape. Not from my parents' home, but from the experience we call life. The intensity of the environment inside my home and the trauma of knowing what lay beyond it all pointed to one harsh conclusion: This world was not a place I wanted to live any longer. And so, I began to plan my suicide.

I considered several methods, but eventually, I settled on one specific strategy: I would jump in front of a truck. It would be quick, and I wouldn't need any special tools or preparation. On several occasions, I put all the grammar and phonics I'd learned to good use by writing a suicide note—a goodbye to my family and to the cruel world I had known for such a short time. I don't know why I never went through with it; those memories, too, are lost to the void. The logs remain empty—years of time I cannot recall.

Not long after that unsettling incident, my family uprooted our lives and moved to Moscow. And again, my memories of that time are like scattered, half-erased sketches—mostly blank, with only a few sharp images cutting through the haze. One of those memories is the suffocating uniform at my new school, with its rough, gray wool scratching against my skin like sandpaper. Another is the image of me, a solitary figure huddled in the corner of the classroom while the teacher leaned in close to my parents, her voice a low, conspiratorial whisper.

"He's a…well…rather *odd* child," she murmured, the words sliding out like a slow-moving poison. I watched my parents' faces as the label settled into their minds—my father's expression hardening like stone, my mother's eyes flickering with a mix of worry and something close to surrender. The judgment in the teacher's voice echoed in the cold, cavernous classroom, where high ceilings and barren walls only amplified my sense of isolation. The other children, their identical gray uniforms blending together like a sea of conformity, seemed part of a world that would never welcome me. I was plump, unathletic, and—as the teacher so clinically diagnosed—*odd.* The tension at home escalated, simmering like a pot about to boil over, while outside, my sense of isolation deepened into a gnawing void.

Then, at fourteen, life yanked me in another direction. We moved again, this time to the United States. And suddenly, everything changed. Within two months, I shot up three inches; within six, I went from fumbling through math problems to tutoring other students. It was as if someone had flipped a switch in my brain—I was awake, alive, and my mind was firing on all cylinders. The sluggish fog that had clouded my thoughts lifted, replaced by a sharp, ravenous hunger for knowledge. Maybe it was the fresh start, the change in scenery, or the different food and air. Whatever it was, I transformed, leaving my old self behind like a snake sloughing off its skin.

But as I evolved throughout my teenage years, the stress and tension at home remained a constant—an ever-present undercurrent. We found ourselves in Chicago, living across from Weiss Memorial Hospital in the free housing they provided. The neighborhood was a far cry from idyllic—adult video stores and porn shops lined the streets, mingling with the strange characters who wandered aimlessly, muttering to themselves or begging for spare change. My father's paltry $4,000-a-year income meant we were scraping by, poor as church mice, always teetering on the edge of poverty.

In the midst of this bleakness, I found my refuge in academics. My mind, now voracious, devoured every bit of knowledge I could find. Books became my sanctuary, the pages my escape. So, when I was offered a surgical residency at Cook County Hospital after I'd finished medical school, it felt like the ultimate triumph, the reward for all my hard-fought battles.

But when I sat down with my mother to share the news, expecting her eyes to light up with joy, I was met with something entirely different.

The moment the words left my mouth, I saw fear and dread creep into her expression. That look was a heavy reminder that even in victory, the past had a way of clinging on, refusing to let go.

"Please, please don't leave. Please don't leave me alone with him." Her voice trembled as she spoke, her eyes wide with fear. She was talking about my father.

"Why don't you just leave?" I asked, desperation creeping into my voice. "Please, Mom. Just get a divorce and be done with this."

But she just shook her head. They'd come too far and endured too much. The years had woven thick, unbreakable bonds between them—maybe not of love or romance, but of hardship, dependency, and trauma. Bonds forged in the crucible of shared suffering. She shook her head again, more slowly this time.

"It's killing me," she whispered, her voice barely audible. "This stress is going to kill me."

I hated to leave her. The guilt gnawed at me, and I would have done anything to stay and protect her, but I was only twenty-four, and my future was just beginning to take shape. My father was a doctor, and she was under the care of a seasoned psychiatrist. What could I do that they couldn't?

Before starting my residency at Cook County, I decided to take a celebratory trip to Mexico—a final breath of freedom before the relentless grind of eighty-hour weeks, sleepless nights, and life-or-death decisions began. I pictured lazy days under the sun, sand between my toes, and maybe a few margaritas. Instead, I ended up in a nightmare that would make any vacation horror story look tame.

The day started like any other on the beach—blue skies, sparkling water, and the smell of sunscreen lingering in the air. I was out swimming, feeling the weight of responsibility melting away for just a moment. But then, out of nowhere, the serene afternoon turned into chaos.

A drunk fisherman, either oblivious or just reckless, plowed his boat toward me, the roar of the engine barely audible over the crashing waves. In a split second, the boat was on top of me, and the propeller tore into my body.

The pain was instant—like a thousand white-hot blades slicing through my flesh, carving deep into muscle and bone. The water around me turned red, thick clouds of blood billowing in slow motion, a stark contrast to the searing urgency flooding my body. My limbs felt sluggish, my strength draining with every passing second, but my mind snapped into focus. *Survive. Stop the bleeding. Stay conscious.*

The boat jerked to a stop. The fisherman loomed over me, his face a mask of shock, his hands trembling, useless. He was watching me bleed out. I didn't have time for his panic. With a last surge of adrenaline, I dragged my left arm out of the water, gritted my teeth, and hauled myself onto the boat's floor. The rough, sunbaked wood scraped against my skin as I collapsed, gasping. My body screamed in protest, but I forced my hands to move—applying pressure, locking down on the worst of the wounds like a human tourniquet.

They say med school prepares you for trauma; I just never expected to be both the doctor and the patient at the same moment. I knew the drill: blood loss is the enemy. My fingers dug into my own flesh, holding back the tide, fighting the darkness threatening to pull me under. Every second mattered. Every heartbeat was a countdown.

By the time they reached the shore, I was barely holding on. My vision blurred, and my breaths came in ragged gasps. Later, they told me I had lost nearly 50 percent of my blood volume; that should have killed me. But my training, my instincts, and my refusal to quit—that's what kept me alive.

I don't remember all the details—trauma has a funny way of blurring the lines between reality and dreamlike confusion—but I vividly recall an eerie sense of detachment, as if I were watching my body from above. Time seemed to stretch, the sounds of the beach and water fading away as my vision tunneled. For a moment, I wasn't in Mexico anymore; I was somewhere else, hovering over my own life, watching the scene unfold like a spectator in a bad movie.

I left Mexico with two hundred stitches, a limp, and a deep, throbbing pain that would take months to fade. It seemed that the legacy of traumatic vacations, a twisted family tradition, had followed me into adulthood. Every time I thought the worst was over, another calamity seemed to be lurking just around the corner. But nothing could have prepared me for what was coming next.

As my body finally began to heal, it was just in time for the punishing demands of my internship at Cook County. From the moment I stepped into the hospital, I was thrust into a relentless cycle of work. Sleep became a luxury I could no longer afford, and I was lucky to get more than two hours a night. It was the rite of passage for all interns: a baptism by fire, or rather, by sleep deprivation and grueling hours. Every young doctor had to endure it, and I was no exception. I pushed through, driven by sheer willpower, as if every stitch in my body was a reminder of what I had already survived and what I was determined to overcome.

Three months later, I got a call. I was deep in the middle of surgery, my hands slick with blood, the scent of iron thick in the air. The operating room was a battlefield that day, but nothing could have prepared me for the war waiting on the other end of the phone.

I raced to my parents' home, adrenaline still surging—but no amount of training, no years of medical school, could have braced me for what I was about to see.

Horror wrapped its vicious tendrils around my entire body as I walked into my parent's home and saw my mother's frail, lifeless form lying on the ground with rope marks around her neck. Overcome and overwhelmed by years of trauma, my mother ended her life. I wanted to run to her, to hold her, breathe life back into her, and tell her that everything would be okay—that we could heal together. But it was too late. She was gone, leaving me with nothing but the cold, brutal reality of her absence. As tears streamed down my cheeks, her desperate words echoed in my mind: *"This stress is going to kill me."*

Grief quickly gave way to a burning rage when I learned that she had tried to hang herself just a week before. She'd failed and somehow convinced everyone around her that it had been a mere accident. But it was no accident. It was a cry for help—a cry that neither my father nor the psychiatrist had taken seriously. She had been under psychiatric care, on prescribed medication, following the so-called "standard medical protocols."

And yet, the system failed her. My family failed her. I failed her. At least, that's what I told myself as I fought to claw my way out of the suffocating fog of guilt, grief, and anger that consumed me after her death.

For months, I was paralyzed by the weight of what had happened. The shock of her loss hit me so hard that I could no longer continue as a surgical resident. The breath was knocked out of me, and I found myself simply existing: going through the motions on autopilot, surrounded by the constant suffering of others. Day and night, I was immersed in a world of trauma and illness, with my father's despondent calls only adding to the darkness that engulfed me.

Two years after my mother's death, I made the difficult decision to leave surgery behind and become an anesthesiologist. At the time, it felt like a step-down choice that lacked the prestige of surgery. But I knew I couldn't sustain the balance needed to complete my residency, not after everything I had been through. The weight of my mother's death, the legacy of inherited trauma, and the suffocating guilt could have easily crushed me.

For a time, they did.

I found myself teetering on the edge, consumed by a darkness that threatened to swallow me whole. The memories of her last words, her desperate pleas, haunted my every thought: *"This stress is going to kill me."*

Those words echoed in my mind, a reminder of the pain she endured and the help I couldn't give her in time. And then, something shifted inside me. All the anger, all the grief, all the disbelief—it all transformed into a fierce drive. What had once been despair now fueled a renewed sense of purpose. Instead of being consumed by that darkness, I made a choice—a choice to fight, to turn my anguish into a force for good. I knew I had to make it through this. I had to survive. And to do that, I needed to find hope. But hope wasn't something that was just going to magically appear—it had to be uncovered, pursued and fought for. The tenacity and resilience I inherited from my parents—born out of years of hardship, survival, and sheer willpower—became the driving force behind that pursuit. Their unyielding spirit propelled me forward, giving me the strength to keep searching for answers, even when it felt like I was wandering through darkness.

As I dove deeper into trauma research, particularly into the workings of the sympathetic nervous system—the primal engine that drives our fight-or-flight response—I started to see the full picture. The more I pressed into the science of trauma, the clearer it became to me that trauma, as devastating as it is, isn't some dark, unknowable force; it's not some mysterious mental condition we can't explain. No, trauma is a natural, physical response—just like a broken bone or an open wound. The body's hyper-alert reaction to stress or danger is hardwired into our DNA for one simple reason: *survival.*

The sympathetic nervous system kicks into gear when we sense danger. It triggers the fight-or-flight response, which floods the body with adrenaline, increases heart rate, raises blood pressure, and gets us ready to move—whether we're fighting a predator or running for our lives. Blood gets redirected from nonessential organs to the muscles and areas that need it most for quick action. This response is built into us, a biological mechanism that has helped humans survive for millennia.

But here's where things start to go wrong. Imagine your fight-or-flight system—the body's emergency response—getting stuck in the "on" position. It's like a car engine revving uncontrollably with no brakes, no off switch. This constant overactivation of the sympathetic nervous system floods the body with stress hormones, leading to a cascade of symptoms: severe anxiety, hypervigilance, paranoia, insomnia, and—in extreme cases—suicidal or homicidal thoughts. This isn't just a psychological problem; it's a physical *injury.* We can see it on advanced brain scans—literal changes in the brain caused by trauma. Trauma, when it embeds itself deep in the body and mind, doesn't just fade away with time. It doesn't quietly recede into the background. Instead, it leaves scars that run deeper than just emotional pain; it alters the very blueprint of who we are.

The conventional approach labels these behaviors and symptoms as a "disorder," but what we're really witnessing is the aftermath of a physical injury to the brain's most primitive systems. This is why I believe the term post-traumatic stress disorder (PTSD) is misleading and fundamentally flawed. What we're really dealing with is post-traumatic stress injury (PTSI)—an injury that can be seen, measured, and (most importantly) treated. It's not about managing a disorder; it's about healing an injury.

Words matter deeply, and this distinction is more than just semantics. Calling it a "disorder" implies that something is inherently wrong with the person—that they are broken in a way that is unfixable. But an injury? An injury can heal.

When you're working with an injury, the goal isn't just to help someone live with it; it's to fix it. With the right treatment and intervention, recovery is not only possible but expected. And this is exactly where the terminology shift becomes crucial. When we mislabel trauma as a disorder, we unintentionally create a mindset that makes people feel like they have to live with the pain forever. That's not the case.

Words can save lives, and words can kill. Misunderstanding the nature of trauma through the lens of an outdated term like "disorder" is not just inaccurate—it's dangerous. It keeps people locked in a cycle of hopelessness. In the chapters ahead, we'll break down why this shift in understanding is so crucial. The words we use shape how we understand trauma, influence the treatments we pursue, and ultimately decide whether someone sees a path to healing or feels trapped in a life sentence.

Imagine you suffered a car accident and broke your leg. But instead of seeking treatment, you felt ashamed of your injury. You spent your whole life limping around, forcing yourself to stand on that broken leg while putting on a brave face so no one would notice. You navigated life with constant pain, doing your best to push through your job, maintain relationships, and engage with the world—not only struggling because of the injury itself but also because of the energy it took to hide the pain. Sure, you took medication to dull it, and maybe even talked to a counselor about the accident, but the injury itself remained. What you really needed was to reset the bone, put it in a cast, and give it time to heal properly. Trauma works the same way: You can cover it up, talk around it, and try to numb it, but without treating the root cause, the wound remains.

This was true for my family. While my father may have come home from war looking physically intact, he carried deep, unseen injuries that marked him for life. These weren't the kind of wounds you could spot with the naked eye, but they were just as real. Sadly, he lived with those invisible injuries for most of his life, and as they went untreated, the trauma spread like a contagious virus, infecting our entire household. My mother and I weren't just bystanders; we became infected, marked by secondary PTSD/PTSI. Trauma, much like a viral illness, doesn't stay contained. It spreads, passing from person to person. My father's unhealed pain infected my mother, who, in turn, was left grappling with her own emotional injuries. The trauma became a sickness that moved from one family member to another, an insidious force that infected us all, keeping the cycle of pain alive.

We live in a world full of people carrying these hidden injuries—people who are trying their best to live normal lives, working, raising children, building relationships—but all while suffering the effects of untreated trauma. These people, like my father, unknowingly spread their pain to others, continuing the cycle. It's like living in a world of untreated illness, where the symptoms are medicated, talked about, but never fully addressed. The implications in society are massive.

Right now, there are children waking up, heading to school with trauma-damaged brains, expected to behave and learn like everyone else. But a brain rewired by trauma is built for survival, not growth or learning. Would you expect a kid with a broken leg to sprint across a soccer field? Of course not. So why do we expect children with trauma to sit still, focus, and thrive in the classroom? Untreated trauma doesn't vanish with time; it takes root, growing deeper.

Kids with trauma grow into adults with trauma, often self-medicating or getting lost in the justice system. It's a vicious cycle, repeating itself through generations. But we now have the science to break that cycle. Trauma isn't a personality flaw—it's a neurological injury.

For far too long, mental health, trauma, and PTSD have been shrouded in mystery, shame, and secrecy. They've been misunderstood and treated as purely psychological problems—something abstract, elusive, and deeply personal. Up until now, talk therapy and medication seemed like the only options for dealing with PTSD/PTSI.

But science is changing the game. We're no longer limited to surface-level fixes—we now have the ability to *actually heal the injury.* We have methods that can break the cycle and reshape how we approach trauma altogether. And I am honored to be at the forefront of this shift, pioneering a breakthrough that is transforming trauma treatment in ways that once seemed impossible.

My breakthrough in trauma recovery has an origin story that might surprise you. It didn't start with trauma at all. In fact, it began in the world of anesthesia and pain medicine.

After losing my mother and stepping into the world of anesthesia, I quickly realized that the field wasn't what I had hoped for. To be honest, I didn't love it. It felt mechanical, routine, detached. But when I shifted into pain management, everything changed. Suddenly, it wasn't just about putting people under—it was about understanding pain at its core, finding ways to stop it, and ultimately uncover something far bigger than I ever anticipated.

It was during this time that my much smarter older brother tossed out an idea that, at first, seemed completely out of left field—using a pain treatment called the stellate ganglion block to help women with hot flashes. It sounded bizarre, but we tried it. And it worked. A procedure I had been using for pain relief suddenly did something unexpected: it erased hot flashes.

That unexpected success opened a door. If this procedure could help with pain and hot flashes, what else might it do? Little did I know, I was on the edge of a discovery that would bring me into the world of trauma treatment. Through a strange series of events (don't worry, you'll get the full story later), I found myself standing at the crossroads between pain medicine and trauma recovery.

At first, the connection seemed unlikely. But as I started piecing things together, the dots weren't just connecting; they were lighting up like a runway, leading me straight to a breakthrough that would change everything.

And that's where things get really interesting. In the pages ahead, we'll dig into how these treatments work, why they're so effective, and how they're capable of healing the brain and body in ways we never thought possible. This isn't just theory—it's already changing lives. Over 10,000 people have used this breakthrough to break free from the cycles of trauma, reclaim their lives, and prove that healing isn't just possible—it's happening.

Take a minute and imagine a world where trauma isn't some invisible curse, quietly passed down through generations like an unwanted inheritance. Instead, it's recognized for what it really is—a diagnosable, treatable injury. A world where people aren't shackled to their pasts, where the weight of old wounds doesn't dictate the course of their lives.

Now, picture the ripple effect. Stronger relationships. Fewer heart attacks. Less cancer. More connected families. Healthier communities. A society no longer drowning in cycles of unhealed pain but rising—because we finally understand that trauma isn't a life sentence.

This is why I'm not just a doctor or a researcher—I'm a Trauma Innovator on a mission to spread hope like wildfire. My North Star? *Trauma isn't a life sentence. It's an injury, and like any injury, it can be treated.* With the right approach, profound and lasting change isn't just possible—it's inevitable.

As a Trauma Innovator, I'm not here to hand out survival tips or teach you how to "manage" your trauma; plenty of books do that already. I'm here to talk about healing in its truest form. This isn't about managing symptoms or learning to live with the pain: it's about rewriting the narrative. Trauma doesn't get to control your story forever. You can reclaim your life, break free from the shadows, and experience a level of recovery that once seemed impossible. Because whether you believe you can or believe you can't—you're right.

This mission isn't just my work—it's my life's calling. It's what fuels me every day, pushing me to bring real, lasting answers to those trapped in the cycle of trauma—just like I once was. I may have a dry wit and a love for a good laugh, but when it comes to this, I don't mess around. Understanding the science behind trauma gave me something I never thought possible: hope. And that same hope? It's what I've dedicated my life to sharing, because I know firsthand how transformative it can be.

Every day, thousands of people are told they have a disorder—a shadow that will haunt them for the rest of their lives. They're told to manage it, to cope with it, as if it's something they'll have to carry forever. I watched my mother live that way. I watched the weight of trauma drain the light from her eyes, watched the system fail her again and again. And that's why this fight is personal.

Because trauma is not a lifestyle. It's not something you just survive with Band-Aids and medication. I've said it before, and you'll hear me say it again (more than once) throughout this book: trauma is an injury. And like any injury, it can be healed.

The real question is—how? How do we heal something that feels so deeply embedded in the very fabric of who we are, including changes imprinted on our DNA? How do we begin to undo the damage, rewrite the patterns, and take back our lives from something that's shaped us for so long? I'm glad you asked, because that's exactly why I'm writing this book. Together, we're going to unravel the mystery surrounding trauma and answer a few crucial questions:

- **What is trauma, really?** Not just the Hollywood version or the worst-case headline, but the quiet, sneaky kind that rewires your nervous system while you're busy surviving.
- **How does trauma live in the body?** Not metaphorically—literally. What does it do to your brain, your immune system, your sex life, your relationships?
- **Who's affected by trauma?** Spoiler alert: it's not just the person who lived through the event. It's the partner, the parent, the child, the friend, the team, the generation.

- **Can trauma be healed—or are we all just supposed to cope forever?** Can we go beyond managing symptoms and actually reset the system?
- **How do these treatments work?** What's really happening in the body—and how do we know it's not just a placebo?
- **What's standing in the way of that healing becoming mainstream?** Who's gatekeeping the cure? And why are we still being handed coping tools when we need recovery blueprints?

In the pages ahead, we're going to pop the hood and dive into the nuts and bolts of how your brain and body really work. We'll break down how trauma injuries ripple through every aspect of life—mental health, relationships, your sex life, and even your lifespan. I'll walk you through the breakthroughs that I and others have made in trauma recovery, including a groundbreaking discovery that's changing lives. You'll meet some incredible individuals I've treated with this new approach, hear their stories, and see firsthand how trauma shaped their worlds—and, more importantly, how this breakthrough transformed them.

We'll also explore the provocative trends in trauma treatment that are strutting onto the scene and showing plenty of leg—like psychedelics and other drugs—and explore whether they're truly helpful or just another distraction. Then, we'll pull back the curtain on the darker forces at play—those systems and power structures quietly panicking, knowing their profits and credibility are on the line as the truth finally comes to light: that there's an affordable, proven path to real, lasting recovery. Buckle up, because it gets a little ugly. My hope is that by the end of this journey, you'll have a clear understanding of what trauma really is, a new perspective on how it affects the brain and body, and—most importantly—a road map to true healing.

Throughout my life, people have often asked me why new breakthroughs in science and medicine, especially in mental health, are so frequently met with resistance, and it's a fair question. Change is hard, especially when it challenges everything we've been taught to believe. Perhaps as you read the pages ahead, you'll encounter some resistance in your own mind, questioning, *"Is this really possible?"* or *"But that's not how it's always been done."* It's natural—we're wired to stick with what we know, even if what we know isn't working.

But here's the thing about pioneers who dare to challenge the status quo—they don't wait for permission. They push boundaries, disrupt comfort zones, and they often make people uneasy. On that note, let me tell you a story about a man who faced resistance of the most tragic kind.

The year was 1846, and our would-be hero was a Hungarian doctor named Ignaz Semmelweis. He was working in the maternity ward of the Vienna General Hospital, and he noticed something alarming: Women in the general hospital were dying at a much higher rate than women in the midwifery clinic. The hospital with three times the death rate was, as you might imagine, staffed by doctors and medical students, while midwives staffed the midwifery clinic and delivered at home. Semmelweis, a young and determined physician, started digging into the data. He ruled out some obvious differences—like the fact that the midwives had women give birth on their sides, while doctors had them give birth on their backs. He even suspected, at one point, that the ringing of a priest's bell when someone died might be scaring the women into a fever. None of this, however, solved the mystery.

Then, something tragic happened: One of Semmelweis's colleagues, a pathologist, pricked his finger during an autopsy on a woman who had died from "childbed fever." He became ill and died with the same symptoms as the women in the maternity clinic.

This was the lightbulb moment: Semmelweis realized that the doctors and medical students were performing autopsies and then delivering babies without washing their hands, transferring deadly "cadaverous particles" from the corpses to the mothers.

Semmelweis introduced the idea of handwashing with a chlorine solution, and the death rate plummeted. He had discovered something monumental—one of the most important breakthroughs in medical history. You'd think this would have been the start of a revolution in public health, right? *Wrong.*

Instead of embracing Semmelweis's findings, many doctors were offended. His theory made it look like they were not only responsible for causing these deaths, but that they were dirty people with unsanitary habits. This was an insult and they rejected it. Semmelweis didn't help his case by berating his colleagues, which only earned him more enemies. The practice of handwashing was not widely adopted at the time, and Semmelweis lost his job. He spent the rest of his life trying to convince doctors to listen, but no one did. He died tragically, fourteen days after being placed in an asylum, possibly from the very infection he had spent his career trying to prevent.

Now, you might be thinking, "What does this have to do with trauma and mental health?" Well, everything.

Semmelweis's story is a cautionary tale about resisting change and ignoring new ideas simply because they challenge the status quo. In the same way that doctors once rejected the idea of handwashing, many people today still resist new approaches to treating trauma and mental health.

We are now on the cusp of a new chapter in mental health, shifting the way we understand, treat, and approach conditions like PTSD/PTSI, suicidal ideation, anxiety, and depression. Imagine the needless suffering that occurred because doctors refused to listen to Semmelweis. Now, imagine the needless suffering that continues today because we are hesitant to embrace new methods of treating trauma.

As you read on, I urge you to keep an open mind. Don't be like the doctors who scoffed at handwashing. Instead, let's push forward, embrace the evidence, and start saving lives. Because just like in Semmelweis's time, the stakes are far too high to resist change.

So, when people ask me how I handle criticism and pushback—because trust me, I've faced plenty as a Trauma Innovator—I often refer to Semmelweis and say, "Well, he was long dead before anyone noticed his life's work." Ironically, twenty years after Semmelweis's death, he was labeled as the "Savior of Mothers." Not a bad legacy, but about twenty years too late.

Fortunately, I'm still here. And while I may not exactly be a young man anymore, I count myself lucky to be alive—and to have the deeply humbling, deeply gratifying experience of seeing lives not just improved, but saved. I'd take that over being ignored for twenty years any day.

My journey, though riddled with pain and loss, led me to a pursuit of answers and breakthroughs that bring real, tangible hope—not the kind of hope that comes from well-meaning platitudes, but the kind that's grounded in science, in evidence, and in the sheer will to live. I could have easily become one of those brooding, introspective souls, forever shadowed by the ghosts of my past, or taken my own life. I could have let the trauma define me, confine me, and reduce me to a casualty of the life I was born into. But I didn't. I refused to let the trauma win. Instead, I channeled all the pain, the anger, and the grief into a quest to understand trauma, strip away the stigma, and bring real solutions to those, like my mother, who have been drowning in their pain with no lifeline in sight.

And so, I invite you to join me on this journey. Together, we'll uncover the truth about trauma, break down the barriers of stigma, and pave the way for a future where hope isn't just a word—it's a reality.

CHAPTER 2
THE FACES OF TRAUMA

What comes to mind when you hear the words "trauma" or "PTSD"? Hollywood has shown us no shortage of intense images: a soldier collapsing on his bed, staring hollowly at the ceiling, lost in the shadows of war; a young woman flinching at loud sounds after escaping abuse; a survivor of a horrific accident jolted awake by haunting dreams. Trauma, in the cinematic world, often appears in sharp, jarring moments—highly visible, intense, and almost theatrical. We're shown characters visibly fractured by their pasts, broadcasting their wounds for the world to see. The message is clear: Trauma is an explosive, life-altering event that wears its scars on the outside. Maybe a soldier cracking under the weight of combat memories, or a victim fleeing some dark alley under the neon of a crime scene? Hollywood's trauma scenes are anything but subtle—think shadows, shaking hands, and lots of close-ups. We're trained to picture trauma as loud and obvious, a dramatic breakdown at the peak of tension. And yet, for most people, trauma doesn't announce itself with flashing lights or a suspense soundtrack. It doesn't always scream. More often, it whispers.

Trauma sneaks in, sits quietly in the corners, and reshapes lives in a thousand subtle and profound ways. It doesn't just exist in those big, cinematic moments—it lingers, weaving itself into the fabric of everyday life, unnoticed but deeply felt. It's the mother who hasn't had a full night's sleep in years, always half-awake, listening for dangers that aren't there.

It's the law enforcement officer scrolling numbly through his phone at the dinner table, his mind trapped in the echo of a call he answered just a minute too late. It's the executive who thrives in high-pressure environments because stillness feels like drowning. It's the person who can't relax, can't let go, can't figure out why they're always on edge.

This is critical to understand because one of the greatest barriers to people seeking help is the belief that their trauma "isn't bad enough." They compare their experiences to extreme cases—combat veterans, abuse survivors, or victims of horrific accidents—and convince themselves that since they haven't lived through something as dramatic, their struggles don't count. But trauma isn't a competition. It doesn't have to fit a Hollywood narrative to be real, and it doesn't need to be extreme to shape the way you think, feel, and move through the world. The truth is that trauma doesn't always wear battle scars or cue dramatic breakdowns. More often, it seeps into a person's thoughts, behaviors, and relationships—altering the way they interact, react, and move through the world until the lines blur, and it's no longer clear what is truly their personality and what is simply an adaptation for survival. It's more than a memory; it's a shift in the nervous system, a rewiring of the brain, a pattern that becomes a prison. These hidden faces of trauma are everywhere, shaping lives in ways so subtle and ingrained that they go unnoticed—even by the person living them.

You see it in the hyperaware friend who never sits with their back to the door, in the child who grows up too fast, in the teacher who seems oddly detached. It's in the overachiever who can't slow down, the parent who struggles to connect, the leader who thrives in chaos but crumbles in peace. Trauma doesn't just affect the individual—it ripples outward, touching families, rewriting generational stories, and shaping entire communities. It embeds itself into culture, into cycles of behavior passed down like an inheritance no one asked for.

In the next two chapters, we're going to tackle the first question: *What is trauma, really?* But before we break it down with brain scans and biology, I want you to meet trauma face-to-face. Not as a concept, but as a lived experience—through heartbeat, story, and raw emotion. You'll be introduced to four remarkable individuals: Michael, Katie, Max, and Trevor. Each one reveals a different facet of trauma and resilience—different roots, different outcomes, but all united by one truth: trauma changes lives. But make no mistake—this book doesn't cast trauma as the hero. We're not romanticizing it or glorifying suffering. We're here to demystify it. These stories show us how trauma can take hold, shape everything...and still not get the final say. After that, we're going to approach the same question from a different angle: by popping the hood. We'll dig into the science—what trauma actually does to the brain and nervous system, how it hijacks the body, and why understanding that mechanism is key to unlocking real healing. By seeing trauma through both lenses—story and science—you'll begin to understand what it truly is, how it operates, and why it matters more than most people realize.

Meet Michael:

Michael was born into a world of chaos. From the moment he opened his eyes, the harsh realities of poverty, neglect, and abuse welcomed him into a cruel world. His earliest memories weren't of lullabies or gentle hugs but of loud arguments, shattered glass, and the feeling of being unseen. His tiny body learned to be quiet, to disappear into corners, hoping not to attract attention. But attention always came, and with it, the sharp sting of a hand or the cold dismissal of being ignored entirely.

His mother was often gone—off chasing her own demons, whether in the form of substances or men who came and went, each more volatile than the last. When she was home, she was distant, lost in her own world of survival, leaving Michael to fend for himself. The cupboards were bare more often than not, and hunger gnawed at his belly, but it was the emptiness in his heart that hurt the most. He was just a boy, but even at five or six years old, he had learned what it meant to feel alone.

His father hadn't stuck around after Michael was born. Sometimes, late at night, his mother would mutter bitter things about the man who had left them, but to Michael, he was just a ghost—an absence as painful as his mother's neglect. Instead, the men who wandered in and out of their small apartment filled the role of the father figure, each one rougher and meaner than the last. They didn't see Michael as a boy in need of care or love: He was just another thing to deal with, another nuisance in a life already full of problems.

The abuse started slowly. At first, it was just harsh words and angry shoves when Michael would accidentally get in the way. But soon, it escalated. His small body became the target for misplaced rage, his cries for help lost in the din of their arguments. His world was one of slammed doors, broken bottles, and bruises that never had time to heal before new ones appeared.

On the worst nights, he'd hide in the small closet in his room, pulling a thin blanket over his head as though it could protect him from the violence on the other side of the door. He learned to hold his breath when the shouting started, hoping that maybe this time it wouldn't end with his door being thrown open, his tiny frame dragged out of hiding for another round of punishment. But more often than not, it did.

His days were no better. Michael would wander the streets near his apartment, dirty and hungry, looking for anything to fill the emptiness. Other kids had backpacks and lunchboxes, parents who walked them to school or picked them up. But not Michael. He was the kid teachers didn't know what to do with—the one who didn't have his homework, who couldn't sit still, who flinched when someone raised their voice. Sometimes, if he was lucky, a kind neighbor might offer him a sandwich or an old toy, but kindness was as fleeting in Michael's world as a sunny day.

The neighbors must have called Child Protective Services dozens of times. Each visit ended the same way—his mother would sweet-talk the social workers, clean him up just enough to avoid suspicion, and send them on their way. And so, the cycle continued.

Until one day, it didn't.

One day, a caseworker arrived and didn't leave. She saw through the facade, through Michael's forced smiles and bruises hidden beneath his shirt. She knew.

That was the day Michael was removed from the only home he had ever known and thrust into the foster care system. As he clutched a garbage bag filled with the few belongings he had, he felt a strange mix of fear and relief. He didn't know where he was going, but at least he wasn't staying. He was out of the fire—at least for now.

But the trauma didn't stay behind. It came with him, stitched into his mind, lodged deep in his heart. By the time he arrived at his new foster home, he was already damaged in ways that no one could see. His world had been one of survival for so long that he didn't know how to live any other way. He didn't know how to feel safe, how to trust, how to be a kid.

The foster system, while created with the best of intentions, wasn't designed to handle boys like Michael. His trauma had rewired his brain in ways that even he couldn't understand. PTSD/ PTSI doesn't show up in children the same way it does in adults. For Michael, it showed up in sudden outbursts, mood swings, and a constant state of hypervigilance. He was always waiting for the other shoe to drop, always on edge. He struggled to sleep, haunted by nightmares that dragged him back to those dark, terrifying nights. He'd wake up screaming, soaked in sweat, his body still trembling from the memories he couldn't escape.

During the school day, his mind was never in the classroom. While other kids were engaged in lessons, his thoughts wandered back to the pain of his past or the uncertainty of what might happen next. His teachers grew frustrated with his inability to focus, constantly annoyed by his fidgeting and daydreaming. He couldn't sit still, couldn't pay attention. His outbursts seemed to come from nowhere, erupting without warning. One moment he'd lash out, the next he would retreat into a shell of silence, unreachable for hours at a time.

The school didn't know what to do with him. They saw only the "problem child" who disrupted the class. He was the constant center of negative attention, labeled "the bad kid," "the dumb kid," "the troublemaker." The patience of those around him wore thin, and even when his foster parents tried to advocate for him, the system seemed to have already made up its mind—he was the kid no one wanted to deal with, a burden rather than a child in need of help.

His bad grades were another constant source of tension. No matter how hard he tried, his mind simply couldn't focus long enough to keep up with the curriculum. To his teachers, he was just lazy, unfocused—a nuisance that couldn't be disciplined into conformity. In truth, he wasn't a bad kid: He was a kid lost in the weight of trauma, but nobody saw that, or (if they did) they didn't know how to help.

What they didn't realize was that Michael's brain had been injured. His ability to learn, to connect with others, to function in a normal setting had been compromised by years of abuse and neglect. This wasn't a case of "bad behavior." Michael's mind had been reprogrammed to survive, not to thrive. Trauma had created a physical injury in his brain, altering the way it functioned. It wasn't his fault, but no one seemed to understand that. Teachers saw a troubled kid; foster parents saw a handful. But Michael wasn't either of those things. He was a boy trapped in a cycle of trauma; his brain unable to break free from the survival instincts that had kept him alive for so long.

Michael's story is one of countless children who suffer from untreated trauma. They're expected to learn, to connect, to function, when in reality, they're fighting a silent war inside their own minds. The world sees them as difficult or disruptive, but what the world fails to recognize is that they're children with injuries—injuries that can't be seen but are no less real than a broken bone.

When Michael walked into my office and sat down, for just a moment, I saw myself in him. He was quiet, plump, and slouched in a way that reminded me of the awkward, unathletic kid I used to be—the kid labeled "odd" by everyone around me, always struggling to fit in. His eyes carried a weight I recognized too well, the same silent plea for understanding that had once been in mine. But little did he know, things were about to change. The treatment we were about to begin would be the first step in a journey that could shift everything for him. Michael's life was on the cusp of something new—a path to healing we'll explore in the pages ahead.

Meet Katie:

Katie was raised by a single mother who wasn't around much. Her mom worked long hours at two jobs just to keep a roof over their heads, and while Katie understood, it left her alone more often than not. By the time she was seventeen, Katie had grown used to feeling invisible. She went to school, came home, and kept to herself. No one really noticed her, and she started to believe she wasn't worth noticing.

Then, she met *him*. He was older, confident, and he took an interest in her when no one else did. At first, it felt like a dream. He made her feel special and valued, like she finally mattered to someone. He'd say all the right things, buy her little gifts, and shower her with attention. For a girl who had always felt forgotten, his affection felt like everything she had ever wanted.

But it wasn't long before the cracks began to show. He had a drug problem, something he kept hidden at first. As his addiction worsened, so did his temper. The sweet words were replaced with sharp insults, the gentle touches turned into rough grabs. Katie wanted to believe it was just the drugs, that the man who had made her feel so loved was still in there somewhere. She thought if she could just love him enough, be patient enough, he'd change back into the man she'd fallen for.

That hope kept her there, even when the violence started. The abuse began subtly. He was charming at first. Attentive. Loving. But over time, the compliments became criticisms, and the kindnesses turned to control. At first, it was small things—a raised voice here, a slight shove there. Nothing too alarming. But then the shoves became pushes, and the yelling became threats. One night, those threats turned into something much darker. She never saw it coming. He was angry, and in a moment, her life shifted. The lines she thought could never be crossed were obliterated. He became violent, and the person she had once loved became her greatest fear.

The physical violence was bad enough, but it was the sexual assaults that left her shattered in ways she couldn't quite comprehend. He didn't just hurt her body—he took something deeper, something she couldn't quite name but could feel missing every day.

For years, Katie stayed. She didn't leave because, like so many others, she felt trapped. He had taken control of everything—her finances, her friends, her sense of self. When she finally found the courage to run, she thought the worst was behind her. But trauma doesn't let go just because you've left the battlefield—it follows you. And for Katie, it followed her everywhere.

At first, it was the nightmares. She'd wake up gasping for air, her heart pounding so hard she thought it might break through her chest. She would find herself drenched in sweat, the sheets tangled around her like a trap. It wasn't just the dreams, though. In the middle of the day, she'd suddenly be transported back to those nights of terror. A sound, a smell, a word—anything could trigger the flashbacks, pulling her back into the suffocating grip of her abuser. She'd freeze, her mind spinning, her body paralyzed as if she were still trapped under his weight.

PTSI/PTSD showed up in ways that made everyday life impossible. It wasn't just the flashbacks; it was the constant hypervigilance. Katie was always on edge, her body tense, ready to react to the smallest threat. Every noise felt like a warning. The creak of a floorboard, the slam of a car door, even a stranger's footsteps behind her—all of it sent her into a spiral of fear. Her body was locked in fight-or-flight mode, always bracing for the next attack, even though she was safe.

And then there was the shame. Society talks about domestic violence and sexual assault, but not enough about what happens afterward. People expect abused people to "move on," to "heal," but they don't understand that healing isn't linear.

For Katie, the shame clung to her like a second skin. She blamed herself for staying as long as she did, for trusting him in the first place. She wondered if others could see it in her eyes—the brokenness, the fear, the ugliness of what had been done to her. Even when she knew, logically, that the abuse wasn't her fault, emotionally, she couldn't shake the guilt.

It showed up in her relationships. Intimacy felt impossible. The mere thought of being touched sent waves of nausea rolling through her. She would become defensive and aggressive at even the gentlest initiations of romantic partners, her body recoiling as if it still belonged to someone else. She wanted to trust again, wanted to feel love and connection, but her body wouldn't let her. It was still in survival mode, still wired to protect her from a danger that no longer existed but haunted her every waking moment.

Her PTSD/PTSI affected her mind, too. She found it hard to concentrate at work. Her thoughts were like static. She became irritable, snapping at friends and colleagues for no reason, pushing people away before they had a chance to get too close. Depression set in, wrapping around her like a suffocating fog. Some days, it felt easier just to stay in bed, to avoid the world entirely. The weight of everything—her memories, her fear, her shame—felt too heavy to carry, but she didn't know how to put it down. She felt disconnected from the people around her, as though her trauma had created a wall between her and the rest of the world. Even in a roomful of happy people who loved her, she felt alone. Friends tried to help, but they couldn't understand. How could they? They hadn't lived it. And Katie didn't have the words to explain what it felt like to carry the weight of her trauma day in and day out.

On the surface, Katie looked like a woman who had "survived," who had made it out. But inside, she was still trapped. Trapped in a body that remembered the violence, trapped in a mind that couldn't forget the terror, trapped in a life she didn't recognize anymore.

PTSD/PTSI had rewired her brain, shifting her into survival mode permanently. It wasn't just a psychological issue—it was a physical injury to her brain, altering how she processed fear, trust, and even love. Every relationship, every social interaction became a minefield, and she walked through life constantly bracing for the next explosion.

When Katie walked into my office and sat down, her body language told me everything I needed to know—shoulders tense, eyes heavy with a pain she had carried for far too long. As we began to talk, I could see the weight of her trauma in every glance, every hesitant word. But when

I explained to her that the injury she'd suffered might not be visible to the naked eye but was a real, physical change in her brain, something shifted. Her eyes filled with emotion, and for the first time, she allowed herself to believe that she wasn't beyond repair. She didn't have to suffer silently, thinking that the world expected her to simply "move on." There was hope for healing that injury. Katie's scars may have been invisible to the naked eye, but they were real, and healing wasn't about forgetting—it was about understanding that she could reclaim her life.

Meet Max:

The first time Max saw his owner, he was just a puppy—small enough to fit in the palm of a hand, his eyes still too big for his face. The man's grip had been rough, his voice low and uninterested.

"Guess you're mine now," he muttered.

Max didn't know what that meant. But he wagged his tail anyway, because that's what puppies do.

The first few weeks were confusing. There was no soft bed, no gentle hands, no warm praise. The man fed him, sometimes, but only when he remembered. Max learned to eat fast because there was never enough. His water bowl stayed empty more often than not. The man didn't speak to him much, except when he was angry—and he was angry often. Max learned quickly: Stay out of the way. Don't make noise. Don't get too close. But no matter how much he tried to be invisible, there were still nights when the man's temper found him. A careless step, a misplaced shoe, and the hand would come down—hard, fast, no warning. The first time, Max yelped in confusion. The second time, he understood: pain was part of life. One day, the man took Max outside and clipped a heavy chain around his neck. It was thick and cold, anchored to a post in the dirt.

"There," the man grunted. "You stay."

And so Max stayed. Days turned to weeks. The chain became his world. Rain soaked his fur. The sun burned his back. He shivered in the cold, curled up as small as he could, waiting for warmth that never came. Sometimes, the man brought food; sometimes, he forgot.

But the worst part wasn't the hunger or the cold—it was the waiting. Every time the man stepped outside, Max's tail thumped against the ground. *Maybe today.* Maybe today would be different. Maybe today, the man would speak to him, play with him, bring him inside. But the man never did. Still, Max waited.

The storm came suddenly—wind howling, rain slamming against the ground. Max pressed himself into the dirt, trying to make himself small. Lightning flashed, and for a moment, he saw everything—the empty yard, the sagging house, the window where the man sat inside, dry and warm. Thunder cracked overhead. Max flinched. Then, with a sharp snap, the chain broke.

For the first time in his life, he wasn't tied down. He stood, unsure, his paws sinking into the wet earth. His body screamed at him to stay—*this is home, this is all you know*—but something deeper, something primal, whispered: *run.* And this time, Max listened.

He bolted into the darkness, paws pounding against the ground, rain stinging his eyes. He didn't know where he was going. He only knew he had to go.

Max ran until his legs gave out. He collapsed beneath the awning of a gas station, his body trembling from exhaustion. He was cold. He was starving. But for the first time, he was free. Morning came, and with it, a voice—soft, curious.

"Hey, buddy."

Max lifted his head. A woman knelt beside him, her eyes filled with something he had never seen before: kindness. She reached out, slow and careful. Max flinched, waiting for the pain. But it never came. Instead, her fingers brushed gently over his muddy fur.

"It's okay," she whispered. "You're safe now."

From that day on, Max had a home—a real one. A soft bed, clean water, meals that came at the same time every day.

But his body still carried the ghosts of his past. Loud noises made him flinch. A sudden movement sent him scrambling for cover. Even when his new owner, Emily, reached out to pet him, he sometimes shrank away before realizing her touch was gentle, not something to fear.

Despite his fear, Max's trauma sometimes manifested in unexpected ways. When cornered or startled by strangers, he would transform—hackles raised, teeth bared, a deep growl rumbling from his chest. These moments of aggression weren't who he truly was, but rather echoes of the survival tactics that had once kept him alive.

At night he would pace in circles, restless, ears twitching at sounds only he seemed to hear. No matter how safe he was, part of him was still waiting for the next blow, the next bad day. Emily saw it all—both his fear and his occasional aggression—the way the past still held him prisoner, and she refused to give up on him. Then came the phone call. My office line rang late one Tuesday afternoon.

"Hello?"

The voice on the other end was tentative but determined. "My name is Emily Clark. I adopted a rescue dog, Max, about three months ago, and I'm…well, I'm struggling to help him."

I listened as she described Max's behavior—the night terrors, the cowering, the unexpected moments of aggression when delivery workers approached the house.

"I've been reading about your work with traumatized animals," she continued, her voice gaining confidence. "The new treatment you've developed. I was wondering…would it be possible to do it on Max?" I could hear the mixture of hope and exhaustion in her voice—the sound of someone who had fallen completely in love with a damaged soul and refused to give up.

"Of course," I replied. "Let's get him in here next week and see how we can help."

The relief in her sigh was audible.

"Thank you," she whispered. "You have no idea what this means to us."

I smiled, though she couldn't see it.

"I think I do," I told her. "And I'm looking forward to meeting you both."

Meet Trevor Beaman:

Trevor Beaman was raised in a low-income neighborhood near Chicago. Trevor's childhood was marked by violence, neglect, and a nightmare that no child should ever have to endure.

From the age of eight, Trevor was sexually molested by his stepfather for nearly a decade. Growing up in a trailer park surrounded by gangs, drugs, and violence, the constant abuse left deep scars on his young mind. His innocence was stolen, and the confusion that came with his body's reaction to the trauma left him questioning everything—was this how all fathers treated their sons?

By the time Trevor reached twelve, the burden of abuse had become suffocating. Nights stretched endlessly as he lay awake, his heart hammering against his ribs at every creak in the hallway. Anxiety circled him like a predator—constant, merciless—while memories of violations played in vivid, technicolor horror behind his eyelids whenever he tried to rest. Eventually, the pain crescendo into something unbearable and Trevor attempted suicide—a desperate bid for an escape that seemed impossible any other way.

Even in the sterile hospital room afterward, his stepfather hovered—all concerned smiles for the medical staff, but eyes that delivered silent warnings whenever they were alone. The man maintained his vigil, ensuring Trevor's silence with practiced precision, coaching him on what to say to counselors and doctors. The very hands that had caused such damage now patted his shoulder reassuringly before visitors, performing the role of concerned parent with chilling perfection. For four more years, Trevor existed in this prison where walls were made of threats and silence. The man who should have been his protector was the architect of his nightmare.

At sixteen, something shifted. A cold realization crystallized: He might not be the only victim. In that moment, fear of silence suddenly outweighed fear of speaking. Trevor finally spoke the unspeakable truth. When his stepfather was in handcuffs, the facade finally shattered.

In the subsequent investigation, Trevor's stepfather confessed to molesting Trevor more than fifty times over the course of six years. The arrest should have felt like freedom. The conviction should have felt like justice. Yet the trauma had embedded itself into Trevor's nervous system, rerouting neural pathways and altering his fundamental sense of safety. The legal conclusion of his abuse was just the beginning of a much longer journey toward healing—one that would follow him through relationships, career choices, and quiet moments for years to come.

Trevor tried to move on. After high school, he earned his way into Purdue University, hoping for a fresh start. He even joined a fraternity, trying to fit into what he imagined was a normal college experience. But the horror movie in his head never stopped playing.

Tragedy struck again when Trevor lost two important people in his life—his best friend to suicide and a former girlfriend to murder. These deaths hit him so hard that Trevor couldn't even bring himself to attend the funeral. The trauma wouldn't leave him alone. The memories in his head were on a loop, no matter how hard he tried to forget them. When Trevor discovered alcohol, it seemed like a solution. Drinking made the memories fade, if only temporarily. But it wasn't a cure: He had to keep drinking to numb the pain, and his life spiraled into a haze of substance abuse.

At twenty, Trevor made a decision that would change his life: He joined the Army. He didn't sign up for glory or adventure; he joined because he wanted to find an honorable death. The idea of dying in service felt more purposeful than the endless suffering he had endured. The structure of the military gave him something to focus on, a way to keep his demons at bay. Trevor became a Green Beret, finding a sense of belonging and purpose in the Special Forces. But while the missions kept him busy, they didn't erase the trauma.

Then, in 2004, Trevor was deployed to Afghanistan. The streets of Kabul felt oddly familiar, like the dangerous streets of Chicago. On every mission, Trevor felt like he was living on borrowed time. Each patrol could be his last. Combat brought new horrors. During one mission, Trevor witnessed an Afghan soldier get blown apart in an instant.

Moments later, his team was ambushed, and a young girl was shot in the head by the Taliban. His team saved her life, but the weight of the violence was crushing. Trevor couldn't process the trauma in the moment. He had to keep going, keep fighting. But the memories of that day, and many others like it, haunted him long after he left the battlefield.

The years of combat deployments, combined with the trauma of his childhood, became too much to bear. Trevor's mind and soul were filled with pain—pain he couldn't escape. Even when he tried to change his life by transferring to Key West to become an instructor, the depression followed him. The weight of his experiences pulled him deeper into despair, and no amount of antidepressants or therapy seemed to help. He described himself as a "walking corpse," a man going through the motions but dead inside.

Then, Trevor and his wife had children, moments that should have been filled with joy and hope. But instead, they plunged Trevor further into depression. Holding his children, seeing their innocence, brought back memories of his own lost childhood. He couldn't stop thinking about the lives he had taken in combat, the parents who no longer had their children because of him. The guilt was unbearable, and he spiraled into a darker place than ever before. Trevor found himself contemplating suicide again. The weight of his trauma, both from his childhood and his military service, was too heavy to carry. He had tried traditional therapies, cognitive behavioral therapy, and medication, but nothing seemed to quiet the horror movie in his head.

Trevor walked into my office carrying the invisible weight of years of trauma. His eyes reflected a man haunted by experiences too heavy to put into words, but buried within that gaze was a flicker of hope—the kind that only comes when someone is desperate for change. He was ready to try something different, something that might finally cut through the fog of hypervigilance and panic. Trevor had heard about a promising treatment—a procedure that could reset the body's stress response and give his nervous system a chance to step off the battlefield. Though skeptical, he was willing to embrace the possibility of relief.

It didn't take long after I treated Trevor for him to notice changes, *big changes,* in the weeks that followed the procedure. The gnawing fear that had gripped him for years loosened its hold, and for the first time in what felt like forever, he told me he could exhale—really exhale. The memories were still there, but they no longer dominated his every thought. Life stopped feeling like a constant state of combat readiness.

This procedure wasn't the end of Trevor's healing—it was the beginning. The fog of trauma started to lift just enough for him to engage with the tools he'd been given in therapy, tools that had once felt beyond reach. He began rebuilding, bit by bit. Suicide, which had once felt like his only escape, was no longer in the picture. Instead, Trevor found himself focusing on the future—on being the father he wanted to be, the husband his wife needed, and the version of himself he thought was lost forever. With newfound clarity, Trevor reconnected with his purpose. He began sharing his story, not as someone defined by his trauma, but as someone who had learned to navigate it, and his voice became a source of hope for other veterans struggling under the weight of unhealed wounds.

There's a reason I wanted you to meet Michael, Katie, Max, and Trevor before we venture into the labyrinth of neuroscience. Their stories illuminate trauma in the theater of everyday life—not as clinical case studies, but as lived experience etched into ordinary Tuesday afternoons and quiet Sunday mornings. And here's the unsettling truth: These narratives echo in countless lives around us. I'd wager that someone in your orbit carries a similar weight—perhaps it's the colleague whose laugh never quite reaches her eyes, the friend who flinches at unexpected touch, or the family member whose anger seems disproportionate to the moment. Perhaps it's even the reflection that meets your gaze in the morning mirror.

When we encounter these stories, something ancient and instinctual awakens within us. Our hearts constrict, our breath changes rhythm, mirror neurons fire as we momentarily inhabit another's pain. This compassionate resonance is our birthright as humans—sacred territory worth honoring. I want you to carry this emotional intelligence forward as we continue, but to braid with it something equally powerful: *radical curiosity.*

Too often we stop at the shores of empathy, offering comfort without pursuing the deeper currents that might lead to transformation. So, let us ask: *What is trauma, beyond its visible manifestations? What mysterious alchemy transmutes one moment of trauma into decades of suffering?* Trauma isn't just psychological impression—it's a physiological revolution, a hostile takeover of our most sophisticated biological systems. Like a master codebreaker that has deciphered our body's encryption, it reprograms neural circuitry, hijacks stress responses, and infiltrates memory storage. It rewrites the very software through which we interpret reality, coloring every incoming data point with the palette of past pain.

Those symptoms we so often dismiss or medicate into submission—the 3 a.m. ceiling staring, the concentration that splinters like thin glass, relationships that wither under inexplicable strain, emotional weather systems that shift without warning, phantom pains that migrate through the body—these aren't character flaws or inconvenient glitches, they're sophisticated warning systems, evolutionary flares launched from the deeper intelligence of your body.

So far, we've examined trauma through the lens of lived experience—the personal stories that reveal its human impact. We've walked alongside individuals navigating its complex terrain in their daily lives. But now, we're going to shift gears and explore what trauma looks like from the angle of science—the neurobiological mechanisms that explain why these experiences manifest as they do.

We've been conditioned to silence these messengers, to treat them as embarrassing interruptions rather than vital communications. In the chapter ahead, we'll decode these signals like linguistic experts breaking an ancient cipher. We'll trace the neural pathways of Michael's emotional numbness, map the autonomic upheaval behind Katie's panic attacks, and illuminate the biochemical cascade that keeps Trevor trapped in vigilance. It's time to reshape shame into understanding, uncertainty into direction, and pain into the starting point of real recovery.

CHAPTER 3
A PEEK UNDER THE HOOD

When we hear the words "trauma," "depression," or "suicide," most of us instinctively tense up. Let's say you're at the Thanksgiving table, innocently reaching for that nearly gray green bean casserole swimming in condensed soup, when your cousin Steph suddenly decides to regale everyone with tales of her shaman's "transformational" trauma-releasing sessions. You can practically feel the collective cringe. People will avoid eye contact, suddenly fascinated with their mashed potatoes, or seize the opportunity to fetch more dry stuffing, just to avoid diving into trauma talk at the dinner table.

Imagine you're at a work lunch and all your coworkers are chatting about their kids' soccer games, Netflix binging, and the latest "life-changing" Peloton class. You decide to open up about something real, something you've been carrying. You tell them that lately, you've been feeling, well, depressed—maybe even dealing with suicidal thoughts. The room goes dead silent. Your coworkers, mid-bite, suddenly freeze. Cheryl from accounting looks like she'd rather talk about her mother-in-law's bunion surgery. Brad from HR nods slowly, like he's not sure if this is a setup, and then blurts out something generic like, *"Well, hang in there!"*

Even with all the progress in mental health awareness, these topics still get the same chilly reception as a forgotten takeout box in the office fridge. People either freeze up, unsure of what to say, or they fall back on well-worn clichés with all the sincerity of a bad Hallmark card.

Now, imagine this: Instead of Cousin Steph launching into tales of her shaman's "life-altering" trauma-releasing sessions, Cousin Brett starts regaling the table with an epic story about how he broke his arm in some "heroic" softball incident. He's hobbling in with a fresh cast, holding up his bruised arm like a badge of honor.

The response? He's showered with hearty claps from the uncles, a laugh from Aunt Carol, and maybe even an extra slice of pie from Grandma for "being so tough." Everyone leans in, asking for every gritty detail, giving Brett the kind of attention usually reserved for family legends.

And let's say instead of confessing that you've been dealing with feelings of depression and suicidal thoughts, you come into work sporting a black eye and a stitched up eyebrow from an "epic" mountain biking mishap.

Suddenly, you're a legend in the office. The boss is asking if you're okay, coworkers want to hear every thrilling detail, and someone's dropping off ibuprofen on your desk. You're practically a folk hero, bonding over battle scars at the coffee machine.

But the moment you reveal a struggle with mental health, you could cut the tension with a butter knife. People look away and the enthusiasm evaporates, leaving behind discomfort and a quick change of subject.

The difference between these scenarios isn't just how people respond, it's a reflection of something much deeper. It demonstrates a startling truth: Most people don't understand what trauma actually *is.* We're comfortable with physical injuries—if Cousin Brett breaks his arm, we get it: it's an injury, something that can be fixed with proper care. But mention "mental health" or "trauma," and people immediately freeze up. Big, spooky words like "disorder," "psychiatry," and "therapy" float around, making us uneasy, as if we're venturing into some dark and mysterious realm.

The reality? Trauma isn't so different from a broken bone—it's an injury. The only difference is you can't see it with the naked eye. But thanks to modern science, we now can see it on brain scans, revealing the physical changes trauma leaves behind—just as real as Cousin Brett's broken arm. There it is: a visible, physical shift in the brain's structure.

Trauma has a very real, physiological impact on the brain and body, influencing our thoughts, our relationships, our sleep, and pretty much every aspect of who we are. And because the injury is internal, people struggle to recognize it. But when we start looking at mental health through the lens of *physiology*, it's like flipping on the lights in a dark room. Suddenly, things make sense.

As a doctor, I learned to view the body pragmatically, through the lens of science. And after my mother's death, it was this steady, logical approach that helped me find solid ground again. Understanding the workings of the brain gave me a framework, a way to reframe trauma as a physiological response, something I could understand and address.

I could dive into the dense terminology—the amygdala, cerebral cortex, dura mater, hypothalamus, occipital lobe, substantia nigra, and so on—but let's be honest: that would probably just make your eyes glaze over. You don't need to pause your life, go to med school, or deep dive into neuroscience. This book is your cheat sheet.

We're going to break down the science of trauma into straightforward language, piece by piece, into something simple and relatable. Because once you get the basics, understanding how trauma impacts the brain becomes a lot clearer, and you'll start to see just how far science has come in redefining what trauma really is.

You've witnessed the impact of trauma in everyday life—now let's explore the "why." This isn't just a new perspective on mental health, it's a revolutionary shift in understanding—a breakthrough poised to redefine how we approach trauma and healing for generations to come.

I want you to picture your brain as a finely tuned engine, a machine that's designed to function in a specific way, with all its gears and pistons firing in sync. When trauma strikes, it's like someone throwing a wrench into that engine. Suddenly, things aren't running smoothly anymore.

Strange noises start, smoke's coming from the hood, and the check engine light is flashing. The system is crying out for help. But here's the problem: Too often, when it comes to mental health, people choose to ignore those warning signs. They don't take their mind to the "shop" to get it checked out. They push through the pain, thinking it'll magically fix itself. Spoiler alert: *it doesn't.*

Once you understand how your brain operates, you can begin to see what's gone wrong—and, most importantly, how to fix it. Instead of wondering why your coworker flipped out over a jammed printer, why you spent an entire night eating cold pizza and binge-watching trash TV, or why you suddenly snapped at a friend for a harmless joke, physiology offers real answers. It shines a light on those seemingly irrational choices that people who've been shaped by trauma often make. And you realize that the check engine light on your car isn't a personal attack on your driving skills—it's just a signal that something's off under the hood.

Think about it. When someone's mood swings from zero to rage in seconds, or when they start isolating themselves from everything and everyone, there's a reason. Even those extreme, dangerous moments—like someone feeling the need to hit 120 mph on the freeway just to "blow off steam"—can be traced back to the body's fight-or-flight system going into overdrive. These responses aren't random: It's the brain trying to survive, even if it's doing so in the worst possible way.

And here's the other thing I love: physiology doesn't lie. Your body is a machine, and like any machine, it follows predictable rules. When those rules are broken—when trauma or stress throws a wrench into the system—the machine starts to malfunction. The brain and body begin to squeak, sputter, and blink at you with warning lights. And if you ignore those warning signs? Well, just like your car, if you don't fix the problem, the whole system can fall apart.

So, before we pop the hood and take a look, let's begin with the fundamental question: *What does the brain actually do?*

Throughout history, humans have come up with all sorts of, let's say, "creative" theories about this. Back in 335 BC, the Greek philosopher Aristotle had an interesting take—he thought the brain was simply a radiator designed to keep the all-important heart from overheating. Imagine that—your brain as a little cooling fan for your emotions. Not exactly spot on, Aristotle, but hey, points for imagination.

Fast forward to around 170 AD, and Greek and Roman physician Galen came up with something a bit more plausible: He suggested that the brain's four ventricles (which are fluid-filled cavities, if you're wondering) were the seat of complex thought and personality. Galen was one of the first people to propose that maybe, just maybe, the brain had something to do with memory, thinking, and, you know, the whole "being human" thing.

Meanwhile, the ancient Egyptians weren't particularly impressed with the brain. They thought it was a useless organ, and when prepping their pharaohs for the afterlife, they'd actually yank it out through the nose with a hooked tool. Picture that for a moment—a hooked instrument, through the nostrils, pulling out bits of brain tissue like it's some kind of leftover spaghetti. And this was an honored process! They were careful not to disfigure the face, of course—*priorities.*

So, in case you missed out on the great scientific breakthroughs of the last few thousand years, let me bring you up to speed: The brain is NOT a radiator, and it's definitely not some useless wet lump to be pulled out of a pharaoh's head like snot. All parts of the brain, in fact, have very specific roles and functions, and trust me, they shouldn't be underestimated.

Take Phineas Gage, for example—a man who is pretty much the poster child for why you should keep your brain intact and fully operational. In 1848, Gage was a railroad foreman in Vermont, going about his business, when an iron rod—over three feet long and weighing more than thirteen pounds—decided to make his skull its new home. In a freak accident, the rod shot straight through his left cheekbone, out the top of his skull, and landed nearly eighty feet away. He was examined in a teaching institution and declared sound because he had normal reflexes and could walk. Miraculously, Gage not only survived, but he was conscious and talking right after the incident.

You'd think having an iron rod rocket through your brain would take you out for good or at least knock a few screws loose, and in Gage's case, it only sort of did. He didn't die and he didn't lose his ability to speak, move, or remember things. But his personality took a major hit. His friends and colleagues said he was "no longer Gage," meaning the guy they knew before the accident wasn't quite the same afterward. Reports claimed that he became erratic, disrespectful, and prone to impulsive, even "animalistic" behaviors. One account even mentioned he started making inappropriate sexual advances at the most improper times—yikes! So yeah, if you ever need proof that all parts of the brain are vital, Phineas Gage is your guy. A word to the wise: Don't go knocking chunks out of your frontal lobe unless you want to start acting like an unruly frat boy.

Let me give you another example. You've probably heard about the Red Baron—a name that's been immortalized in countless books, movies, and war stories. Manfred von Richthofen, aka the Red Baron, wasn't just a legend: He was a real person, a top German fighter pilot during World War I, and the most feared flying ace in the skies. Known for his scarlet-colored plane and unmatched precision, Richthofen became a symbol of mastery in aerial combat. But beneath the myth, the Red Baron's story gives us another fascinating glimpse into the brain's inner workings.

Manfred von Richthofen was a legend—a brilliant tactician in the air, known for his sharp mind and precise coordination, taking down eighty Allied planes in dogfights. But the Red Baron's legendary skills were put to the test in July 1917 when, during a dogfight, he sustained a serious head injury. A bullet tore into his skull, leaving him with blurred vision and compromised consciousness. Despite his severely impaired state, Richthofen somehow managed to land his plane safely. Imagine that for a moment—his brain had taken a direct hit, yet parts of it were still functioning well enough to bring him down to the ground. His cognitive abilities may have been impaired, but other brain functions kicked into gear to ensure his survival. Even with his mind struggling to stay alert, his motor skills, spatial awareness, and the ability to land a plane remained intact.

Now, what do these stories have to do with our bigger conversation? They show just how crucial every part of the brain is in keeping us operating at our best. These examples remind us that the brain isn't just a mysterious lump in your skull—it's a finely tuned, interconnected machine. Each part has a role to play, and when one piece falters, the rest can either compensate or crumble. Understanding how the brain works isn't just fascinating—it can literally be the difference between life and death.

We now know that the brain is far more than a lump sitting in your skull (sorry again, Egyptians!). It's a three-pound marvel, an intricate network of neurons, blood vessels, and cells that run the big show we call the human experience. The brain is made up of parts that work together like a well-oiled machine—a complex, high-powered control center that governs everything you do, think, feel, and experience. It doesn't just keep you alive; it makes you who you are. Thought, memory, emotion, touch, motor skills, vision, and breathing—every process that regulates your body runs through this command center.

Now, if you were to slice open your brain (not literally, let's leave that to the neuroscientists), you'd find a structure made up of 60 percent fat, with the rest being water, protein, carbs, and salts. The brain isn't a muscle, but it works hard like one, constantly firing off electrical signals and sending chemical messages through billions of neurons. These neurons—those hardworking little nerve cells—make sure everything from your breathing to your most vivid memories is processed and stored.

When I was in medical school, neuroscience felt overwhelming. Too many structures, too many functions—it was like trying to memorize an entire city's subway system in one night. But over time, I realized that understanding the brain doesn't have to be complicated. If we're talking about trauma, you only need to focus on four key players:

1. **The Neocortex**—Rational Thought and Decision-Making
2. **The Limbic System**—Emotion and Memory Processing (all mammals are the same here, by the way)
3. **The Amygdala**—The Brain's Threat Detection System (this is the part of the limbic system that is responsible for rage and fear)

4. **The Brainstem**—The Body's Survival Engine

Each of these plays a critical role in how we process trauma, react to stress, and, ultimately, how we heal.

1. The Neocortex—Rational Thought and Decision-Making

The neocortex is the newest and flashiest part of the brain—literally. "Neo" means new, and "cortex" means outer layer, making this the high-tech control center responsible for logic, reasoning, problem-solving, and planning. It's where all your deep thinking happens. For trauma, the prefrontal cortex (PFC)—a part of the neocortex—is the real MVP. This area allows you to analyze situations, regulate emotions, and override impulsive reactions. It's the part of your brain that lets you pause before flipping off the guy who just cut you off in traffic.

Want to flex your PFC? Studies show that playing video games like *Super Mario Bros.* can engage this area, and cognitive therapies that stimulate the PFC can help regulate emotions in trauma survivors. But here's the kicker: When your amygdala senses danger, it can hijack the whole system—overriding the PFC and shutting down your ability to think clearly. If your PFC is strong enough, it can keep the amygdala in check. But if the amygdala is running the show, logic and calm go out the window—and that's when the real problems start.

2. The Limbic System—The Emotional and Memory Hub

The limbic system is responsible for processing emotions, forming memories, and regulating motivation. It is present in all mammals, meaning the emotional wiring of a rat, a dog, and a human share many similarities. One of the most important structures here is the hippocampus—named after its resemblance to a seahorse (*hippocampus* means "horse sea monster" in Greek). The hippocampus is crucial for memory formation, organization, and context processing—it helps your brain recognize that past threats are no longer present.

In trauma survivors, the hippocampus can become dysregulated, making it difficult to distinguish between past and present danger. This is why individuals with PTSD/PTSI may experience flashbacks or intrusive memories—the brain struggles to properly file traumatic experiences into the past, so they feel like they're happening right now. Damage to the hippocampus has also been linked to memory impairments. In extreme cases, such as after a stroke, individuals may struggle to form new memories at all. Studies have shown that activating the hippocampus—through therapies involving structured memory recall and spatial navigation tasks—can help people with PTSD/PTSI regain control over their trauma responses. You can actually *build up* your hippocampus by playing *Tetris.* No, really—brain scans back this up. The game's focus on visual-spatial processing stimulates the hippocampus, and a stronger hippocampus can help regulate and even suppress the amygdala's overactive fear responses. So, the next time someone tells you video games are a waste of time, just tell them you're working on your trauma recovery.

3. The Amygdala—The Brain's Threat Detection System

The amygdala is the fear and threat detection center of the brain. It plays a key role in detecting danger and initiating the body's fight-or-flight response. When faced with a perceived threat, the amygdala triggers a cascade of physiological reactions, preparing the body to respond. This rapid-response system is essential for survival—if you see a car speeding toward you, you need to jump out of the way before you have time to logically process the situation.

One fascinating study found that removing the amygdala in rats prevented them from developing PTSD, but while this isn't a viable solution for humans, it does go to show just how important the amygdala is.

4. The Brainstem—The Body's Survival Engine

The brainstem is the oldest and most basic part of the brain, in charge of keeping you alive. It controls things you don't even have to think about, like breathing, heart rate, and digestion. But when the amygdala senses danger, it sends a distress signal to the brainstem, kicking your body into survival mode. And that's where things get interesting.

To see how all these systems work together, imagine you're walking alone at night when suddenly, footsteps echo behind you. Your body tenses. Your heart pounds. You don't stop to think—you just feel the surge of adrenaline, your senses sharpening, your muscles coiling, ready to sprint. That's your brain's emergency response system kicking into action. The moment something scary, dangerous, or just plain freaky happens, your eyes send signals to the thalamus—your brain's sensory relay station. The thalamus, like an air traffic controller, decides where to send the incoming information. Now, it has a choice:

> Send the data to your neocortex—the logical, thinking part of your brain, where you can calmly assess the situation.
>
> Bypass logical thinking and toss the information straight to the amygdala—your built-in panic button.

I think you already know the answer.

In a moment of danger, the amygdala doesn't wait around for logic. If you're about to be hit by a car, you don't have time to analyze the physics of impact—you just jump. The amygdala slams the emergency button like a contestant on a game show, instantly triggering the fight-or-flight response before your thinking brain even knows what's happening.

In much the same way, your amygdala is wired to override the slow, logical neocortex and take charge when your brain thinks you're in danger. Sure, sometimes it overreacts (like when you scream at the printer), but that's only because it's built to keep you alive—not to ask questions. Deep in the brainstem, the locus coeruleus—your body's stress accelerator, the seat of fight or flight—roars to life, flooding your system with norepinephrine, adrenaline's slightly less famous but equally intense cousin.

Your heart races, your lungs expand, your pupils dilate, and your digestion grinds to a halt—because when survival is on the line, digesting your lunch isn't exactly a top priority. At the same time, the hypothalamus activates the HPA axis (hypothalamic-pituitary-adrenal axis), unleashing cortisol, the body's primary stress hormone. Unlike norepinephrine, which acts instantly, cortisol keeps you on high alert for longer—ensuring you stay ready for action even after the initial adrenaline rush fades.

The moment this happens, your heart starts pounding, and your brain shuts out all unnecessary thoughts and functions. Blood vessels in places that aren't essential—like your intestines, fingers, or (let's just say it) between your legs—constrict, while blood rushes to your muscles to fuel your escape. It's your body's way of saying, *"No time for distractions, Don Juan!"* because, let's face it: this is no time for romance. When you're running for your life, foreplay is off the table.

Your entire system is now primed for survival. Meanwhile, your neocortex—your rational brain—is still booting up, metaphorically sipping its coffee, trying to figure out what the hell just happened. This lightning-fast response is why humans have survived for thousands of years. It's a brilliant system—when it works correctly.

Even after you've escaped whatever danger you were in, your body doesn't just instantly calm down. You're still breathing hard, heart racing, adrenaline surging. Your brain keeps pushing norepinephrine through your system, keeping you on edge for a while longer—just in case that danger comes back. It's this feedback loop—an ancient survival mechanism—that locks you into that heightened state.

The problem is, for some people, their brains get stuck with that panic button jammed down, keeping them in constant fight-or-flight mode even when the danger is long gone. It's like the body keeps expecting a lion to jump out from behind every corner, even when they're just standing in line at the grocery store. And that, my friend, is where things start to go haywire.

When the fight-or-flight system stays locked in high gear for too long, or the stress is intense enough, your body starts making changes that make it even harder to power down. This state of "sympathetic overdrive" is driven by elevated levels of nerve growth factor (NGF), which sparks nerve sprouting—yes, actual nerve growth. This means more sympathetic nerves come online, ramping up norepinephrine production throughout your brain.

And here's where it gets really interesting: the nerves in your neck, specifically through the stellate ganglion (think of it as the railway station for fight-or-flight signals between your spine and brain), start sprouting new pathways. These pathways keep norepinephrine levels elevated, trapping you in high alert. It's like your entire system gets rewired for survival mode, creating a vicious feedback loop that makes switching off the alarms nearly impossible.

I call this the "Danger Loop." Once you're stuck in it, it's like your brain's panic button is held down, keeping you on edge, even when the threat is long gone. Your fight-or-flight system doesn't care about context—it's designed to react, and after enough hits, it stays in overdrive.

This happens because NGF acts like fertilizer for your sympathetic nerves, encouraging growth and laying down new pathways that keep the system running at full throttle. The more these pathways develop, the harder it becomes to switch off survival mode, leaving you stuck in a perpetual state of readiness for danger that may never come.

Every surge of panic or anxiety isn't just a reaction—it's reinforcement. The longer you remain in the Danger Loop, the more your brain and body adapt to maintain it. It's like digging a trench: at first, it's shallow, easy enough to climb out of. But with every panic attack, every anxious moment, that trench deepens, becoming harder to escape. Over time, the fight-or-flight system becomes more powerful and automatic, tightening its grip. Rather than just feeling anxious or uneasy, your body is actively building a more efficient system to keep you stuck, making it more challenging to return to calm.

The truth is that trauma—regardless of whether we label it "big" or "small"—can set off a cascade of biological changes that hijack the brain's sympathetic nervous system, pushing it into overdrive. This isn't something you can just willpower your way through or "snap out of." It's not a mindset problem—it's a physical reaction, a biological process happening deep inside your brain.

This overactivation isn't visible to the naked eye, but believe me, it's there—clear as day on advanced neuro scans. The amygdala, which is responsible for processing and generalizing fear, lights up like a fire alarm in individuals with PTSD/PTSI, showing far more intense reactions to emotional triggers compared to those without trauma. Even chronic stress leaves a mark—animal studies have revealed structural changes in the amygdala itself, with neurons sprouting tiny spines, reinforcing fear pathways like deep grooves worn into a record.

If you were to remove the amygdala, PTSD/PTSI simply wouldn't exist. Let that sink in. The evidence is measurable, physical, and undeniable. It's not only in your head; it's in your brain.

By now, you can probably see why calling it "post-traumatic stress disorder" doesn't quite fit. As I've said before—and will say again—this isn't a disorder. It's an injury, a biological wound, not a permanent scar you're doomed to carry forever. But living with the effects of an untreated injury? That's a different story. As you've seen in the stories I've shared, trauma left unaddressed doesn't just fade into the background—it shapes lives, warps relationships, and hijacks futures. And unless we understand it, treat it, and heal from it, the damage compounds, bleeding into every aspect of life.

Now, you've gotten to see trauma through two lenses: the raw, lived experiences of real people, and the cold, clinical science happening under the hood. It's not reserved the dramatic Hollywood version or the worst-case headline. It's the quiet kind that embeds itself while you're just trying to make it through the day. The kind that hijacks your nervous system without ever announcing itself.

Now, it's time to answer the next question on our list: *How does trauma live in the body?*

What does it do to your brain, your heart rate, your immune system, your sex life, your relationships? How does a survival response meant to protect you end up running your entire life without your permission?

In the next chapter, we're cracking that wide open.

CHAPTER 4

WHEN YOUR BODY REMEMBERS WHAT *YOU* TRY TO FORGET

We've already seen how trauma hijacks the nervous system, rewiring the brain and trapping you in survival mode—but what if I told you it goes even deeper? Trauma doesn't just live in your head. It wears down your entire body—DNA to bloodstream, cell by cell, system by system—breaking you down from the inside out. This isn't just a mental battle: Trauma doesn't politely stay in the brain like a bad memory tucked away in a dusty corner, it floods the entire system. It compromises your biology. And, if left unaddressed, it quietly steals years off your life. The body and mind are connected, after all. That's why we have a neck—not just to keep your head from rolling off, but to remind you that what happens in your brain doesn't stay in your brain...it travels south.

The relationship between trauma and physical health remains one of medicine's most overlooked connections. While we've grown more comfortable discussing the psychological aftermath of trauma, we rarely confront its physical toll: weakened immune function, chronic inflammation, cardiovascular strain, digestive disruption, and even accelerated cellular aging. This isn't speculative science—it's documented across decades of research spanning diverse populations from war veterans to abuse survivors. The evidence forms an undeniable picture: Trauma doesn't just change how you feel—it fundamentally alters how your body functions at its most basic levels.

Trauma and the Immune System: A Silent Sabotage

Let's start with the immune system—the body's built-in defense force. Think of it as your personal security team: fast, responsive, always scanning for threats, ready to neutralize whatever bacteria, virus, or rogue cell dares to mess with you. Under normal circumstances, that system works beautifully. A pathogen shows up, the immune team responds. Threat resolved? It stands down and goes back on patrol. But when trauma enters the picture, that well-oiled machine starts to malfunction.

Here's why: Trauma doesn't just shake you emotionally—it locks your nervous system into a constant state of emergency. Your fight-or-flight engine—the sympathetic nervous system—was designed for short bursts of action: a quick getaway from danger, or a sudden need for vigilance. Once the threat passes, the parasympathetic nervous system (aka rest-and-digest mode) is supposed to take over and bring everything back to baseline. But trauma doesn't play fair. It doesn't just pull the alarm—it breaks the switch. Your body stays on high alert long after the danger is gone, as if the threat is still right there in the room. It's like someone duct-taped the gas pedal to the floor and threw away the brakes. And when that happens? Your immune system pays the price.

In this locked on state, your body is flooded with stress hormones like cortisol and adrenaline. These chemicals are incredibly useful in short bursts—think sprinting from a bear or lifting a car off someone in a crisis. But when they're constantly circulating? They become toxic.

Elevated cortisol:

Suppresses the immune system. Your white blood cells—the soldiers of your defense squad—start to malfunction. They become sluggish, disorganized, or even go rogue and attack healthy tissue (hello, autoimmune diseases).

Promotes inflammation. Cortisol initially reduces inflammation during acute stress, but in chronic stress, your body starts ignoring the signal. It's like your cells develop stress hormone deafness. The result? Unchecked, low-grade inflammation that simmers in the background and wrecks long-term health.

Interferes with tissue repair and healing. Your body prioritizes short-term survival over long-term maintenance. So, you get slower recovery times, more illness, and higher susceptibility to infections and disease.

Ever wonder why some people seem to catch every cold that goes around? Why they're always tired, dealing with weird joint pain, unexplained rashes, or mystery diagnoses that seem to float in and out of doctors' offices without resolution? They're not weak. They're not making it up. They're not broken. They may be carrying trauma.

Their immune systems are trapped in a loop they didn't choose and can't shut off. Their bodies are trying to survive a threat that's no longer there—but the nervous system never got the memo. And while they may look fine on the outside, internally they're fighting a war they didn't sign up for.

The worst part? Most of them don't even know it. They've just been told they're "sensitive," "stressed," "out of balance," or that it's "all in their head." But it's not—it's in their hormones, their immune response, and their biology. And until we start treating trauma as the full-body, full-system injury that it is, we're going to keep missing the real cause—and keep mislabeling millions of people as anxious, lazy, or sick...when what they really are is **stuck in trauma misery.**

Inflammation: The Fire You Don't See

Trauma fuels chronic inflammation—the quiet arsonist setting slow-motion fires all over your body. It doesn't come in loud, waving red flags. It sneaks in, lights the match, and kicks back while your immune system scrambles, confused and exhausted, trying to keep the blaze under control. We're not talking about feeling "a little run down." We're talking about serious, chronic conditions—the kind that slowly drain your energy, wreck your mood, and, eventually, land you in the hospital: heart disease, type 2 diabetes, obesity, autoimmune diseases, fertility issues, gut disorders, chronic fatigue, and even certain cancers. What do they all have in common? Inflammation. And trauma is a master at keeping that flame alive. Here's what the science says: people with PTSD/PTSI or long-term trauma exposure tend to have sky-high levels of inflammatory markers—stuff like:

- CRP (C-reactive protein): Think of it as your body's internal flare gun. When CRP levels are high, your system is sending a clear distress signal—something's not right. The good news? This is a common blood test you can ask your doctor to check.
- IL-6 (interleukin-6): A key player in your immune response, but when it overstays its welcome, it's linked to everything from depression to insulin resistance.
- TNF-α (tumor necrosis factor-alpha): The name says it all. This one's involved in cell death and inflammation and is a big player in autoimmune and degenerative diseases.

These aren't just abstract lab numbers—they're your body's way of telling you it's stuck in a loop, a loop where it never fully powers down. Where the immune system—dysregulated and overactive—is still firing on all cylinders long after the threat has passed. And when the body's on high alert all the time, guess what it stops doing well? Repairing. Resting. Regulating. That's why trauma survivors often feel like they're breaking down in slow motion. One week, it's gut issues; the next, joint pain. Then comes the brain fog, the fatigue, the mystery inflammation that doctors can't quite explain. This is what happens when the Danger Loop runs the show. The body stops prioritizing long-term maintenance and shifts into survival mode—permanently. This inflammatory state doesn't just make you feel miserable—it actively shortens your lifespan, as measured by epigenetic clocks, increased disease risk, and higher rates of heart attacks. It lays the groundwork for major disease. It compromises immunity, increases pain sensitivity, and literally accelerates aging. We're not being dramatic here, we're being biological. Your body isn't failing you. It's responding exactly how it was designed to in the presence of ongoing danger. The problem is the trauma turned the danger switch on—and then broke it off.

PTSD: The Hidden Catalyst for Heart Disease and Cancer

PTSD/PTSI doesn't just haunt the mind, it wages a silent war on the body, acting as an unseen catalyst for severe health conditions like heart disease and cancer. Extensive research highlights a compelling link between PTSD and cardiovascular diseases. Individuals with PTSD face a significantly higher risk of developing heart-related ailments. A study involving over 8,000 veterans revealed that those with PTSD had a nearly 50 percent greater risk of developing heart failure over a seven-year period compared to their non-PTSD peers. This association underscores the profound impact of psychological trauma on heart health. While the relationship between PTSD and cancer is complex, emerging studies suggest a potential link. Chronic stress and PTSD can lead to immune system dysregulation, creating an environment conducive to cancer development. Although more research is needed to establish a definitive connection, the existing evidence highlights the importance of monitoring cancer survivors for PTSD symptoms and addressing them promptly.

PTSD and Premature Death: The Data Doesn't Lie

If all of this feels heavy, it should. Because we're not only talking about feeling "off" or having a few bad days. We're talking about real, measurable, life-shortening consequences—ones that show up in the most brutal of statistics: *lifespan*. A 2015 meta-analysis published in *The American Journal of Geriatric Psychiatry* found that individuals with PTSD faced a 29 percent higher risk of death from all causes compared to those without the condition. The risk was even greater for those with severe or untreated PTSD.[1]

Other research has echoed these findings, linking trauma to significantly higher risks for cardiovascular disease, cancer, and neurodegenerative disorders like Alzheimer's. But it goes deeper—literally, to the level of your DNA.

A study involving twins revealed that those with current PTSD were "epigenetically older" than their non-PTSD counterparts by an average of 1.6 to 2.7 years. This is called DNA methylation age acceleration—essentially, trauma flips certain genetic switches that speed up your biological clock. And yes, this can actually be measured. In a study conducted by the US Department of Veterans Affairs, researchers followed 241 trauma-exposed veterans and discovered that those exhibiting hyperarousal symptoms of PTSD showed accelerated DNA methylation aging—a biological shift associated with a 13 percent increased

---

1 Lohr, J. B., Palmer, B. W., Eidt, C. A., Aailaboyina, S., Mausbach, B. T., Wolkowitz, O. M., Thorp, S. R., & Jeste, D. V. (2015). Is Post-Traumatic Stress Disorder Associated with Premature Senescence? A Review of the Literature. American Journal of Geriatric Psychiatry, 23(7), 709–725. https://doi.org/10.1016/j.jagp.2015.04.001

risk of death over [2]a 6.5-year period.[3] Even veterans receiving regular care through the VA are dying younger—often by decades. And that's without even factoring in the twenty-two to forty-five suicides happening every single day. Chronic trauma wears the body down. It weakens the immune system, accelerates cellular aging, and traps the body in a constant state of low-grade inflammation. And if that's not enough to get your attention, consider this: a meta-analysis published in *BMC Psychiatry* reviewed multiple studies and found that individuals with PTSD had a 47 percent higher overall mortality risk, and a 32 percent increased risk of earlier death compared to people without PTSD.[4] Let that sink in.

Trauma doesn't just steal your peace of mind—it steals time, vitality, and quality of life. It speeds up the aging process from the inside out and leaves you stuck in a cycle of invisible misery that wears you down long before your time. Unless we start treating it like the full-body injury it is, we're going to keep losing people long before their time. Let me be blunt: trauma kills. Not just metaphorically, not just emotionally: biologically, systemically, quietly. One of the most haunting things about trauma is that your conscious mind doesn't even need to remember it for your body to suffer. Childhood trauma, developmental trauma, attachment injuries—they can all create lifelong immune dysfunction, often without a single flashback or obvious sign of PTSD. You might not even know why you're always sick, always tired, always anxious. But your

---

2 Wang, Z., Hui, Q., Goldberg, J., Smith, N., Kaseer, B., Murrah, N., Levantsevych, O. M., Shallenberger, L., Diggers, E., Bremner, J. D., Vaccarino, V., & Sun, Y. V. (2021). Association between posttraumatic stress disorder and epigenetic age acceleration in a sample of twins. *Psychosomatic Medicine, 84*(2), 151–158. https://doi.org/10.1097/psy.0000000000001028

3 Erika J. Wolf, Mark W. Logue, Tawni B. Stoop, Steven A. Schichman, Annjanette Stone, Naomi Sadeh, Jasmeet P. Hayes, and Mark W. Miller, "Accelerated DNA Methylation Age: Associations With Posttraumatic Stress Disorder and Mortality," *Psychosomatic Medicine* 80, no. 1 (January 2018): 42–48, https://doi.org/10.1097/psy.0000000000000506.

4 Dinuli Nilaweera, Aung Zaw Zaw Phyo, Achamyeleh Birhanu Teshale, Htet Lin Htun, Jo Wrigglesworth, Caroline Gurvich, Rosanne Freak-Poli, and Joanne Ryan, *BMC Psychiatry* 23, no. 229 (April 2023), https://doi.org/10.1186/s12888-023-04716-w.

cells know. Your immune system knows. The body remembers—even if you don't.

This chapter isn't here to scare you—it's here to wake you up. Because here's the hope: Your body can heal. Neuroplasticity and physiological reset aren't just buzzwords—they're the real deal. Treatments now exist (that's what this book is ultimately about) that don't just help you *manage* trauma, they help you unwire it at the level of the nervous system itself. When you interrupt the Danger Loop, calm the cortisol chaos, and finally reset the sympathetic system, the results are nothing short of transformative. Your immune system begins to repair itself. Inflammation cools down. Your body recalibrates. Energy comes back online. Sleep returns. Digestion improves. You stop catching every virus within a thirty-foot radius. In other words, people don't just feel better—they come back to life. Even sex can actually be fun again.

The truth is that sometimes you can't deep-breathe or green-smoothie your way out of trauma, not entirely, because trauma doesn't just live in your mind: it lives in your chemistry, in your bloodwork, and in your cells. But here's the good news: If trauma can turn the heat up—we can learn how to turn it back down. And that's exactly where we're headed. I've devoted my life to a treatment that doesn't just manage trauma—it initiates a full-body reset that's already changing lives around the world. But first, while we're answering the question "How does trauma live in the body?", there's one more effect hiding behind the curtain—a consequence that trauma experts seem to mysteriously forget to mention in their TED Talks. PTSD/PTSI has a nasty habit of sabotaging something that should be joyful, connective, and—let's be honest—capable of generating enough electricity to power a small city. Got a guess?

Here's a hint:

What do Marvin Gaye's silky vocals…Patrick Swayze's hips in *Dirty Dancing*…and that suspiciously cozy mountain cabin with a bearskin rug have in common?

That's right—sex.

I know, I know—this started as a cerebral deep dive into trauma and neuroscience, and now we're slipping into the most intimate room of the house. Maybe you're raising an eyebrow. Maybe you're wondering where exactly this is headed. Maybe you're giving this page the kind of look reserved for a plot twist you didn't see coming. But don't bail now—stay with me. Because what happens in the bedroom is one of the clearest mirrors of what trauma does to the body. And if you're scratching your head wondering what trauma and brain science have to do with the bedroom, trust me—you're not alone. But when it comes to trauma's grip on the body, the bedroom might just be ground zero.

CHAPTER 5

FIGHT, FLIGHT, OR FOREPLAY

In all my years working with folks who've been through some of the toughest battles—elite soldiers, first responders, survivors of all sorts of unimaginable situations—there's one symptom of PTSD/PTSI that hits a little different. Sure, the hypervigilance, the jumpiness, the sleepless nights—they're awful. But when trauma starts throwing a wrench into the bedroom? That's when things really hit home. For a lot of people, the "battlefield" that hurts the most is the one where they've lost their edge in…well, you know, *the sack.* Spoiler alert: nobody's happy.

Let's start with something surprising—did you know that over 80 percent of combat veterans struggle with some form of sexual dysfunction directly linked to their trauma?[5] And here's the kicker—only about 15 percent of these cases ever improve on their own.[6] We're talking thirty-five-year-old men who should be in their sexual prime. This isn't just an unfortunate "side effect" of aging or general health issues: This is trauma rewiring the body, disrupting one of the most personal and

5 Kenneth A. Hirsch, "Sexual dysfunction in male Operation Enduring Freedom/Operation Iraqi Freedom patients with severe post-traumatic stress disorder," *Military Medicine* 174, no. 5 (April 2009): 520–522, https://doi.org/10.7205/MILMED-D-03-3508.

6 V. Gruden and V. Gruden Jr., "Libido and PTSD," *Collegium Antropologicum* 24, no. 1 (June 2000): 253–256, https://pubmed.ncbi.nlm.nih.gov/10895553/.

essential aspects of life. And that's exactly what happened to my good friend, Scott Greyson.

Scott Greyson was the kind of Marine who could disassemble an M16 blindfolded and navigate through enemy territory using just stars and instinct. Three tours in Afghanistan had earned him a chest full of medals and the unwavering respect of his unit. He'd survived firefights where the air itself seemed to burn, pulled bleeding comrades from collapsed buildings, and kept his cool when an IED turned his convoy into twisted metal just six feet behind him. But stateside, the war followed him home in ways no one had prepared him for.

The Rusty Nail wasn't Scott's usual haunt, but the thunderstorm had driven him into the first shelter he could find. He claimed a corner stool, back to the wall—old habits—when she walked in.

Lisa shook rainwater from her umbrella, her scrubs still visible beneath her unzipped jacket. Her shoulders carried the unmistakable weight of a twelve-hour hospital shift, but when the bartender called her by name, her exhausted smile transformed her face entirely.

"The usual, Lisa? Rough one today?"

"Lost a kid in the ER," she said quietly, slipping onto a stool two spaces from Scott. "Some days I wonder why I became a trauma nurse."

Scott found himself sliding a bowl of pretzels toward her. "Because you're the kind of person who can handle the worst days and still come back tomorrow," he said, surprising himself.

She looked up, really seeing him for the first time. Something in her gaze told Scott she was assessing him with the same clinical precision she probably used on patients—noting his rigid posture, the tension in his jaw, the careful distance he maintained.

"Sounds like you know something about that," she replied.

Their first date at Vincenzo's felt like stepping into another life. Candles flickered across her face as she told stories about the patients who'd recovered against all odds.

For the first time in months, his shoulders relaxed. The hypervigilance that had kept him scanning rooftops and doorways faded into the background as he found himself leaning in, captivated by the way her hands—capable hands that had literally held beating hearts—moved when she spoke passionately.

"You're different," she said, reaching across the table to touch his wrist.

The electricity of that simple contact shocked him. His body remembered desire, remembered connection—a feeling so foreign after years of emotional numbness that it was almost painful in its intensity.

Later, in the privacy of his apartment, as her lips found his and her hands traced the scar along his collarbone, something catastrophic happened. His body, which had responded to commands flawlessly through the worst conditions imaginable, simply...shut down. The desire remained trapped in his mind while his body refused to participate.

"It's okay," Lisa whispered. "Really."

But it wasn't. Not to Scott.

He tried again the following weekend—a carefully orchestrated evening at the Skyline Lounge where everything was perfect. The sunset painted the city gold, a saxophone crooned in the background, and Lisa looked at him with such warmth that it physically ached.

Yet when they returned to his place, history repeated itself with cruel precision. This time, shame crashed through him like an incoming mortar. He'd navigated minefields with steadier hands than these that now trembled as he made an excuse about early morning appointments. Scott's phone rang for days afterward. Each time Lisa's name appeared on the screen, he stared at it until the ringing stopped. Eventually, the calls did too.

It wasn't just Lisa. Scott systematically dismantled every potential for intimacy. He declined invitations, fabricated emergencies, and perfected the art of friendly-but-distant. Each retreat reinforced the battlefield logic: avoid situations where failure is guaranteed.

The isolation grew like a cancer. Nights stretched longer. His apartment, once a sanctuary from the chaos of deployment, became a cell where he served time for a crime he couldn't name. The man who had once led others fearlessly through gunfire couldn't now lead himself into vulnerability. The irony wasn't lost on him—he'd survived bullets and bombs, only to be undone by the prospect of tender touch.

What haunted Scott most wasn't the dysfunction itself, but the growing certainty that some essential part of his humanity had been left behind in the dust. The capacity for intimacy—physical and emotional—that made life worth living seemed as distant as the stars he'd once used to find his way home.

PTSD/PTSI doesn't just steal your peace of mind—it seeps into every corner of your life, even the most personal. For Scott, it felt like losing a piece of himself, a part that no amount of grit, discipline, or bravado could restore. I've worked with enough hardened warriors to know that, if given the choice, many would rather lose a limb than lose their ability to connect in the bedroom. Because let's be real—that's one battlefield where no one wants to feel powerless. The heartache here cuts deep. Many of these veterans and first responders would sooner run into gunfire than admit to this kind of vulnerability. Their partners feel confused, hurt, even rejected, while these warriors feel trapped—reaching for connection but finding their bodies unresponsive. And it's not relegated to veterans. Trauma doesn't discriminate: whether it's childhood trauma, intimate partner violence, or neglect, the scars can show up in ways that go far beyond flashbacks and anxiety.

But why? What exactly hijacks the brain when the lights dim and intimacy beckons? How does a sophisticated defense system—evolutionarily perfected to save your life—become the saboteur of your most primal connections? The answer lies in a neurobiological perfect storm where survival circuitry collides catastrophically with our capacity for pleasure. Remember the moment we looked under the hood to see what happens when the body senses danger? Heart pounding, oxygen flooding the muscles, digestion grinding to a halt. It's not chaos—it's coordination. The amygdala takes control, overriding higher brain functions to run a single program: survive.

Now, imagine that same system activating in the bedroom. Here's where norepinephrine enters the picture—your body's chemical version of an alarm bell. At low levels? No desire. At moderate levels? Great sex, strong connection. But at high levels—especially the chronic high levels seen in PTSD—desire vanishes.

When PTSD/PTSI takes hold, it transforms your sympathetic nervous system into a hypervigilant sentry that never sleeps. Picture an aircraft carrier's combat alert system perpetually blaring, every system primed for immediate threat response. Spectacular for evading predators in the Paleolithic wilderness; catastrophic for modern intimate encounters. Here's the neurophysiological cascade: Your brain's emergency protocol kicks in. *Redirect blood flow to major muscle groups? Executed. Flood system with catecholamines? Complete. Elevate heart rate, tension peripheral muscles? Mission accomplished.* Everything deemed non-mission critical—including the intricate vascular mechanics of arousal—gets shut down. After all, the biggest sex organ is the brain, and when the amygdala takes over, it biochemically vetoes desire. It's like your hypothalamus is broadcasting: *"Procreation protocols suspended! Survival parameters not met!"*

This is the merciless biology of trauma: your entire system locked in physiological red alert. Blood that should engorge erectile tissues or trigger vaginal lubrication is commandeered for quadriceps and cardiac muscle instead. Your autonomic nervous system treats sexual arousal like requesting in-flight meal service during an airplane crash. The insidious complexity deepens: that relentless cortisol cascade—alongside norepinephrine and adrenaline—creates a neurochemical environment fundamentally incompatible with intimacy. Your external presentation might project calm, but internally, your neuroendocrine system is executing emergency protocols. So precisely when vulnerability should feel safest, your body's alarm system screams: **"AMBUSH IMMINENT!"**

The hypothalamus is the key part of the brain responsible for sexual arousal—responsible for initiating the neurochemical processes behind sexual arousal in both males and females, though its role in male arousal is particularly well-documented. But when the amygdala is overactivated, it can suppress hypothalamic activity, reducing desire and shutting down the drive for intimacy.

This isn't psychological reluctance. It's autonomic physiology operating exactly as designed. Which means it responds not to talk therapy alone, but to interventions that directly address the dysregulated nervous system beneath conscious control. I know all that doctor-speak can get a little complicated, so when I need to explain it to a practical, no-nonsense, give-it-to-me-straight kind of guy, I just say:

> *"Think about it—your body is smart. It knows that you don't want anything 'sticking out' while you're running from a tiger. That could seriously reduce your chances of survival."*

That one seems to stick. (Pun fully intended.)

This misfiring system doesn't just affect romantic moments—it impacts relationships, self-esteem, and the ability to connect deeply with others. Trauma rewires the brain's survival system, leaving little room for connection, warmth, or vulnerability. And the deeper we dig into its effects, the clearer one thing becomes: trauma doesn't just affect the person who lived through it—it spreads. Which brings us to a bigger truth—one that might hit closer to home than expected. At this point, we've looked at trauma through two powerful lenses: the raw, lived experiences of real people and the cold, clinical science unfolding beneath the surface. We've answered a major question: *How does trauma live in the body?* Now we arrive at the next one: *Who's actually affected by trauma?*

And maybe, just maybe, you're thinking, *"This is all fascinating... but I'm not sure it applies to me—or anyone I love."*

I hear you, truly. But I'd ask you—gently—to pause. Because here's the truth: this conversation absolutely applies to you. Whether you've lived through trauma, love someone who has, or simply exist in this messy, beautiful, unpredictable world—you are affected. Unaddressed trauma isn't confined to therapy rooms or war zones; it shows up in boardrooms, classrooms, bedrooms, and dinner tables. It rewires how we parent, how we lead, how we protect, how we connect—and most of all, how we love. It shapes the way we see ourselves. It dictates how we treat others. And it silently controls how we cope when life throws us sideways. This isn't just about *survivors.* It's about all of us. Understanding trauma isn't an intellectual exercise. It's not a "mental health thing." It's a survival skill, a leadership skill, a parenting skill, and a relationship skill.

It's the missing piece in almost every room where humans struggle to perform, connect, or feel whole. So, before we dive into the revolutionary breakthroughs in healing, I want you to hold onto this one truth: this book isn't just for "them." It's for you. Because once you understand trauma—truly understand it—you start seeing the world, your relationships, and yourself with entirely new eyes. And that kind of clarity? It changes everything.

So, about our next question: "Who's actually affected by trauma?" The answer might be bigger—and closer to home—than you think.

CHAPTER 6

IRON MAIDEN OF THE MIND

At thirty-four-years-old, David Allen should have been in the prime of his life, yet every day felt like a battle he was losing. Once, he had been proud of his role as a combat medic—a man trained to heal, to save lives in the midst of chaos. But now, those same skills and instincts that had made him a steady hand in the storm seemed powerless against the turmoil within him. Twice deployed to Iraq, first from 2006 to 2007 and then again from 2009 to 2010, David had been thrust into the heart of the conflict, witnessing humanity at its darkest. He had faced the brutal realities of war head-on, surrounded by violence, bloodshed, and the unimaginable loss of life. The things he had seen, the things he had done—they had etched themselves into his mind like scars that no passage of time could heal.

David had once been the savior, the one who ran toward the injured when everyone else sought cover, the one who tried to hold the line between life and death. But now, despite all he had done for others, he couldn't save himself from the battles raging within his own mind.

The nightmares started after his first deployment—vivid, relentless dreams that dragged him back to the desert every night, where the echoes of explosions and the cries of the wounded filled his mind. No matter how hard he tried, he couldn't escape the horrors that haunted him, replaying them in an endless loop in his mind. During the day, it wasn't much better. The memories would invade his thoughts without warning, overwhelming him with images and sensations that left him reeling. Crowded places became unbearable, the noise and movement too much for his frayed nerves. The anger—sudden and uncontrollable—was always simmering beneath the surface, ready to explode at the slightest provocation.

His wife learned to navigate his moods, but his children didn't understand. One day, his son decided to play an innocent game, trying to sneak up on his dad and make him jump. But David's combat reflexes, honed in the chaos of war, took over before he even realized what was happening. In a split second, he grabbed his son's arm with tremendous force. The sickening crack of his son's arm breaking under his grip was something he would never forget. That was the day he realized just how deeply the war had embedded itself, how it had morphed him into something he no longer recognized.

The medications hadn't helped. Each new prescription—citalopram, buspirone, sertraline, Prozac, Wellbutrin, Minipress—offered a fleeting glimmer of hope that quickly faded as the symptoms persisted, unchanged. Therapy felt like a broken record, the same conversations, the same lack of progress. He was drowning, and no one could throw him a lifeline.

Then, four months after his second deployment, the weight of it all became too much to bear. The arguments with his wife, the guilt over his son, the unrelenting nightmares—it all came crashing down.

In a moment of utter despair, David made a decision. He filled the bathtub with hot water, sat down, and picked up the razor blade. The pain was sharp, but it was nothing compared to the torment in his mind. He watched as the water turned red, the warmth of the bath seeping into his skin, numbing him, pulling him under. He had hoped it would be quick. He had hoped it would be quiet. But his wife came home earlier than expected.

The next thing David saw was the bright lights of the emergency room amid the frantic voices of doctors and nurses. He had failed again, but this time, it was a failure that brought him back to the harsh reality he had tried so desperately to escape. David was admitted to inpatient psychiatry at Tripler Army Medical Center. Within those sterile walls, he had no idea what would happen next, no idea if there was any way out of the hell he was living in. All he knew was that he couldn't go on like this. Something had to change, but what?

A few weeks later, David found himself sitting in a doctor's office. His eyes were hollow, the look of a man who had given up hope, someone resigned to living as a prisoner in his own mind. He had tried just about everything—medications, therapy, the works—yet nothing had given him more than a fleeting break from the nightmares and anxiety. But this time, he'd heard about something different—a treatment with an unconventional approach to trauma, a procedure that promised more than just managing the pain.

The question gnawing at him was simple but heavy: Could this really work? Could this be his way out of the darkness that had swallowed him whole for so long? Or was it just another false glimmer of hope in a long line of disappointments? Sitting there, in that sterile room, David wasn't sure he had enough left to keep looking for answers if this turned out to be just another dead end. But he knew he had to try.

We're going to press pause here at this critical moment. David's story, as you'll see in the pages ahead, is far from over. What happened next changed everything for him, and the treatment he received is unlike anything you've heard before. But I'm not going to reveal the breakthrough just yet—because before we dive into the science behind it and how it works, we need to take a step back for a reality check.

The conversation we're having about trauma isn't a casual one. This isn't the kind of thing you can skim through and forget about. It's urgent, it's pressing, and it's life-altering for those trapped in the same dark places David once was. So, before we go any further, we need to make sure we're all on the same page, grounded in the reality of what's at stake here.

When we think of trauma, stories like David's often come to mind—military veterans, rape survivors, victims of domestic violence. These are the individuals who have faced what I sometimes refer to as BFT, or big f--king trauma. Yes, you heard that right, and yes, I coined that very precise medical term myself. BFT refers to those catastrophic, soul-crushing experiences that leave deep, jagged scars. Now, why do I use that term? It's because trauma exists on a spectrum. There's your everyday stressors, there's what is commonly referred to as PTSD, which stems from significant but singular traumatic events, and then there's CPTSD (complex PTSD), which comes from repeated and sustained trauma. But then, there's the far end of the spectrum is extreme trauma—or what I refer to as BFT.

BFT is when you're not only hit by trauma, you're steamrolled by it—repeatedly. It's the kind of horror that leaves you feeling like a prisoner, your life held hostage by the relentless, inescapable memories. Imagine being chained to a sink and raped for ten years—that's BFT. David's story falls into this category. It's extraordinary, even in its darkness. The horrors he's faced are the kind that most of us can only imagine, and, thankfully, never have to endure.

As a doctor devoted to trauma and pain management, I've also heard more horrific stories than I care to count—stories that could rival the most insidious plotlines that Hollywood could dream up. And while these stories are tragically more common than they should be, they still represent only a minority of trauma cases. The majority of people won't face BFT in their lifetimes, and that's a good thing.

But here's the reality check: Trauma, in all its forms, is far more pervasive than we often acknowledge. It's not just the Davids of the world who come close to ending their lives because of it. Trauma isn't always about the big, life-altering events. Sometimes, it's the accumulation of smaller wounds that can be just as devastating, just as paralyzing. Take my mother, for example. She didn't go to war. She wasn't the victim of some headline-making tragedy. But the pain she carried was real—and it led her to end her life. Because here's what people often miss: the severity of trauma doesn't always predict suicidal ideation.

The truth is, conversations about suicide and mental health aren't just important—they're urgent. Now more than ever, they're necessary. This isn't just about improving the quality of life; it's about saving lives. I hate to be the bearer of bad news, but there is a suicide crisis unfolding, and it's far closer to home than most people realize. Suicide isn't just a distant statistic or something that happens to "other people." It's a devastating reality that's not far from anyone's life. This is a subject that's both deeply personal and alarmingly widespread, touching more lives than we might dare to acknowledge. This crisis is here, in our homes and communities, and it's not something we can afford to turn away from anymore.

So, before we dive deeper, we need to face some hard truths head-on. I urge you—don't stop reading, don't look away, and don't skim over what you're about to read. Stay with me, because what follows is more than just numbers. These figures represent real people, real lives, and real pain. They're a stark reminder of why this conversation is so desperately needed.

Operation Deep Dive, an ongoing research project sponsored by America's Warrior Partnership (AWP), finds that the true rate of self-inflicted deaths among service members is twice as high as the oft-quoted statistic of "twenty-two deaths a day" reported by many veterans' groups. Deep Dive estimates that as many as forty-four veterans die each day from suicide and other self-inflicted means, including drug overdoses, officer-involved shootings, high-speed single-driver fatal traffic accidents, accidental gunshots, and drownings.[7] There are many different sources that place this number anywhere between twenty-two and forty-five, but the truth is that even one is too many. These men and women survived war zones only to lose the battle on their home turf.

And they're not alone. Suicide rates among US preteens have been climbing steadily, increasing by 8.2 percent annually from 2008 to 2022[8] after a brief period of decline. Just think about that—preteen kids, who

---

7 America's Warrior Project. "Operation Deep Dive Summary of Interim Report," Dataset for 2014–2018. Accessed June 30, 2025. https://docs.house.gov/meetings/VR/VR00/20220929/115166/HHRG-117-VR00-Wstate-LorraineJ-20220929-SD001.pdf.

8 Donna A. Ruch, Lisa M. Horowitz, Jennifer L. Hughes, Katherine Sarkisian, Joan L. Luby, Cynthia A. Fontanella, and Jeffery A. Bridge, "Suicide in US Preteens Aged 8 to 12 Years, 2001 to 2022," *JAMA Network Open* 7, no. 7 (July 2024): e2424664, https://doi.org/10.1001/jamanetworkopen.2024.24664.

should be worrying about homework and playground squabbles, are instead grappling with thoughts of ending their lives.

Unfortunately, this extends beyond veterans and preteens. Suicide rates across the United States have been on a steady rise over the past two decades, making it a serious public health crisis. In 2017, fourteen out of every 100,000 Americans died by suicide, according to the CDC's National Center for Health Statistics. That might seem like just a number, but it represents thousands of lives—each one a story cut tragically short. What's more alarming is that this rate reflects a 33 percent increase since 1999,[9] reaching the highest age-adjusted suicide rate recorded in the US since 1941. And just for a little historical context, the last time we saw rates this high was during the Great Depression and the beginning of World War II.[10]

More recent data paints an even grimmer picture. In 2022, the provisional number of suicides in the US was 3 percent higher than the final total number of suicides in 2021.[11] A study published in the *British Journal of Sports Medicine* analyzed National Collegiate Athletic Association (NCAA) athlete deaths from 2002 to 2022 and found that suicide has become the second leading cause of death among college athletes, following accidents. The research also revealed that the proportion of deaths by suicide doubled over the two decades, increasing from 7.6 percent in the first ten years to 15.3 percent in the second ten years.[12] According to the CDC's WISQARS Leading Causes of Death Reports for 2022, suicide was the eleventh leading cause of death overall in the United States. It was the second leading cause of death among individuals aged ten to fourteen and twenty-five to thirty-four, the third leading

[9] Holly Hedegaard, Sally C. Curtin, and Margaret Warner, "Suicide Mortality in the United States,1999–2017," National Center for Health Statistics Data Brief, no. 330 (November 2018), https://www.cdc.gov/nchs/products/databriefs/db330.htm.

[10] Leah Kuntz, "A Year of Record-High Suicide Rates," *Psychiatric Times* 41, no. 4 (April 2024),https://www.psychiatrictimes.com/view/a-year-of-record-high-suicide-rates.

[11] Ibid.

[12] Bridget M. Whelan, Stephanie A. Kliethermes, Kelly A. Schloredt, Ashwin Rao, Kimberly G. Harmon, and Bradley J. Petek, "Suicide in National Collegiate Athletic Association athletes: a 20-year analysis," *British Journal of Sports Medicine* 58 no. 10 (April 2024): 531–537, https://doi.org/10.1136/bjsports-2023-107509.

cause among those aged fifteen to twenty-four, and the fourth leading cause among those aged thirty-five to forty-four. To put it in perspective, there were nearly twice as many suicides as homicides in the United States that year.[13]

If all these stats feel overwhelming, here's the bottom line: Every day, twenty-two to forty-four veterans die by suicide, preteen suicide rates are increasing by over 8 percent each year, and for college athletes, suicide is now the second leading cause of death. I know, this is heavy stuff. But we need to talk about it because these aren't just numbers: These are people—sons, daughters, friends, and loved ones—who felt that the pain of living was too much to bear. I know that feeling. This should be one of the greatest points of focus for the medical and psychiatric communities right now. We need answers on *why* this is happening and—more importantly—why it's getting worse.

But there's one big issue we need to address—a major barrier that's standing in the way of real progress. And it involves you.

The unfortunate reality is that most people dealing with suicidal ideation hide it, often because of the overwhelming stigma that surrounds it. This stigma isn't just confined to the individual; it extends to their families and society. A husband might not want people to know his wife is suicidal, or a mother might go to great lengths to hide her teenager's struggle. And it's not just familial pressure—there's also personal and societal pressure. People fear being judged, labeled as weak, or seen as broken. The fear of being perceived this way forces many to keep their struggles hidden, treated like a black sheep rather than someone in need of help.

Another part of the problem is the widespread belief that only BFT causes suicidal ideation. The reality? All types of PTSD/PTSI—whether from combat, childhood neglect, toxic relationships, or any other form of sustained stress—can lead to suicidal thoughts. These days, we're constantly exposed to other people's trauma—through Netflix documentaries, crime series, social media, and viral stories on the internet.

---

13 "Suicide," National Institute of Mental Health, accessed June 30 2025, https://www.nimh.nih.gov/health/statistics/suicide.

And while this has raised awareness, it's also created a kind of "trauma flexing"—an unspoken hierarchy where people compare their suffering: *His trauma is bigger than yours. Her pain is more valid than his.* This kind of thinking is dangerous because it convinces people that if they haven't been through BFT, their trauma must not be "real" or "serious enough" to warrant help.

That mindset needs to change—because it's keeping far too many people suffering in silence. Conversations about mental health issues and suicide are still pushed into the shadows and shrouded in shame. They are treated as a moral failing or a weakness of the mind. But think about it—no one judges another person for having a broken leg. We don't tell them to "just walk it off" or "toughen up." Yet when it comes to an injured mind, the response is often very different. Far too many people believe that those struggling with suicidal thoughts just need to "get over it," "toughen up," or "stop obsessing." This harmful mindset not only silences those in need of help but also prevents them from seeking the support they desperately require.

On this note, I want to give you a somewhat vivid metaphor that I often use to describe those struggling with mental health issues and suicidal ideation.

In the Middle Ages, there was a torture device called the iron maiden. Imagine this: a human-shaped box, its interior lined with sharp iron spikes. The victim would be forced inside, and as the door shut, the spikes would drive into their body, not deep enough to kill instantly, but just enough to cause slow, agonizing pain. The spikes were strategically placed to avoid vital organs, ensuring the person bled out over time, suffering every excruciating moment. The iron maiden was designed to prolong the torment, keeping the victim trapped in a horrific state of living death.

Now, imagine what it would be like to live inside an iron maiden—not in the physical sense, but in the mind. This is what it feels like for someone struggling with suicidal ideation. It's not iron spikes piercing their body, but instead, it's the relentless spikes of self-degradation, shame, guilt, fatigue, fear, pain (both psychological and physical), self-loathing, overwhelm, and the slow erosion of hope. Each of these emotional spikes digs in deeper every day, causing pain that's just as real and just as unbearable as any physical wound. But unlike the iron maiden of the Middle Ages, where others inflicted the torment, the iron maiden of the mind is a self-contained prison. The spikes come from within, and the victim is left to suffer in silence, often feeling as though there is no escape.

The iron maiden of the mind doesn't just inflict pain randomly, it follows a brutal sequence. It starts with self-degradation and self-loathing, the first spikes that pierce through, opening wounds that bleed shame and guilt. These emotions aren't just psychological—they're deeply physiological as well. Western science often likes to compartmentalize—treating the brain as separate from the heart, the lungs, the kidneys—but in reality, they're all interconnected. You can't separate the two. The mind influences the body, and the body reinforces the mind, creating a vicious cycle that feels impossible to break.

When your mind is consumed by self-loathing, your body reacts. Your fight-or-flight response, controlled by the sympathetic nervous system, kicks into high gear. Fear and anxiety flood your system, preparing you to confront danger. But when the danger is within your own mind, there's no escape, no resolution—just a constant, unrelenting state of alertness. This ongoing state of hyperarousal drives up levels of cortisol, the body's stress hormone. And while cortisol is helpful in short bursts, keeping us sharp and responsive, chronically elevated levels are toxic. They lead to fatigue, insomnia, and an ever-deepening sense of overwhelm. The spikes of fear and pain become relentless, dragging you into a state of exhaustion. Sleep becomes elusive, leaving you trapped in a cycle of wakeful torment. This is where the iron maiden truly does its damage—it doesn't just cause pain, it wears you down until all that's left is the overwhelming desire for an end to the suffering.

Einstein once said, *"Talking to a beautiful woman for an hour feels like a second. Sitting on a hot plate for a second feels like an hour."* And I while can personally confirm the first part—time does fly when you're in good company—the hot plate part? Well, I'll take Einstein's word for it. But that's precisely the experience of being trapped in the iron maiden of the mind. The pain makes every moment stretch into an eternity, turning seconds into hours, hours into days. Being trapped in an iron maiden of the mind makes every single day feels like an uphill battle. You feel drained of all energy, will to live, and *hope*. The iron maiden isn't just a metaphor for emotional pain, it's a description of how that pain becomes a physiological prison, where each aspect of your being is under siege. This is why breaking the stigma around suicide is so important. We need to recognize the deep, interconnected processes that trap people in this cycle and start offering the comprehensive support that's truly needed.

When I interviewed veterans who had attempted suicide, many of them said the same haunting thing: *they didn't want to die forever—they just wanted to die for a little while.* They just wanted a little relief.

I hope you're thinking back to that peek under the hood we took—how it revealed the deep physiological changes trauma imprints on the body. For far too long, we've treated mental health and suicidal ideation as purely psychological, overlooking the very real physiological effects that create an iron maiden of the mind and body—trapping people in pain they can't escape. Understanding this is crucial because it proves why we can't reduce suicidal thoughts to just a "mental" issue. It's a full-body assault—a relentless loop of suffering that deserves the same urgency and compassion as any physical injury.

So, let's circle back to David's story from Chapter 6 for a moment, because everything we've discussed in the previous chapter explains why his life had become a minefield, even after he left the physical warzone behind. David wasn't just haunted by the horrors of his combat experience; his brain and body were trapped in the Danger Loop—a constant state of high alert that he couldn't escape from, no matter how hard he tried. His amygdala, the part of his brain that's supposed to keep him safe in a life-or-death situation, had gone rogue. It was stuck pressing the panic button over and over again, flooding his system with norepinephrine and locking him into survival mode.

Every loud noise, every sudden movement—it all sent his brain spiraling back into the chaos of war. His sympathetic nervous system, through the stellate ganglion, kept pumping out stress signals like they were still on the battlefield, even though he was safe at home. And the longer this cycle continued, the deeper those neural pathways became. His body was essentially growing new nerves, powered by nerve growth factor, reinforcing the Danger Loop.

When David snapped and broke his son's arm in a reflexive, tragic moment, it wasn't just the result of lingering emotions—it was the direct consequence of a brain that had rewired itself to see danger in everything. His amygdala, his brain's security guard, had taken over, acting before his conscious mind even had a chance to catch up. This also explains why the therapy, the medications—none of it worked. Because David wasn't just dealing with emotional trauma; he was dealing with a full-blown physiological reprogramming. His brain had changed at a fundamental level, locking him into the Danger Loop and making it nearly impossible for him to calm down, to feel safe, or to just *be.*

David's suffering wasn't just psychological—it was deeply physical. His brain wasn't "broken," but it had been rewired by trauma to prioritize survival at all costs, even when there was nothing left to survive. His fight-or-flight system, designed to protect him in moments of danger, had taken over completely, running on autopilot and forcing his body to stay in high alert long after the real battles had ended.

And that's the cruel reality of the Danger Loop—it traps you. It's like a faulty alarm system that keeps blaring, even though the fire has been put out. Until David could break that cycle, until he could find a way to hit the reset button on his amygdala and sympathetic nervous system, his mind and body were going to continue waging wars against ghosts of the past. His body, locked in that overdrive state, was stuck bracing for threats that were no longer there.

The danger loop doesn't let you sleep—and that alone can push someone to the edge. Chronic sleep deprivation isn't just exhausting; it's a known risk factor for suicide.

This is why David's existence was like living inside his own version of the iron maiden—imprisoned in a mental and physical cage, spiked by fear, anger, and pain at every turn, with no way to escape. But now, with everything we've discussed, you can see why it's isn't a matter of "getting over it" or "learning to relax." His brain had been rewired in a way that simply couldn't be undone by sheer willpower. David needed something more than just coping mechanisms. He needed a full reset—a way to break free from the Danger Loop and finally step out of survival mode once and for all.

Any conversation about mental health and suicide has to start with empathy—a deep, genuine understanding of just how critical this issue is. It's not only about those who've experienced extreme trauma; it affects everyday people, children, and teens—those waking up each morning, trapped in their own mental prisons, unsure how to survive another day. The greatest step to breaking the cycle? *Hope.* Hope is what unlocks the door, the force that shifts the question from *"Can I keep going?"* to *"Is healing possible?"* Without it, the weight of trauma feels inescapable. But with it, even the darkest moments can become the beginning of something new.

If you're dealing with suicidal thoughts, you need to give yourself some grace. If you know someone who is struggling, you need to approach them with care. This isn't some distant issue that happens to "other people." The reality is, someone in your family, friend group, or community is likely facing it right now. It's on all of us to educate ourselves, challenge outdated beliefs, and dismantle the stigma that keeps so many suffering in silence. That's why the treatment we're about to discuss is so critical—because it's redefining the entire conversation around trauma and how we heal from it.

There's a quote by Max Planck that says something along the lines of: *"Science advances one funeral at a time."* In other words, progress often only happens when the old ideas die with the people who held them. But we can't afford to wait for that anymore. We can't stand by while the "old guard" clings to antiquated methods, resistant to new breakthroughs. And it shouldn't take the loss of your son, daughter, spouse, or friend for us to finally wake up and push for real change. Too many people are walking around inside their own iron maiden of the mind, trapped in a cycle of pain and despair. We can't let the establishment's grip on archaic thinking stand in the way of saving lives.

The good news is that we don't have to. We have the tools, right now, to break this cycle—to free those trapped inside and to start saving lives before another name becomes a statistic. Science is offering us the key to unlock the iron maiden of the mind—even for people like David, who may feel that all hope is lost.

So, it looks like you stuck with me through this last chapter, and I'm happy about that. I know it was pretty heavy stuff—probably a lot to digest—and it's haunting, I know. But we're past all the spikes and torture chambers, and we've pulled back the curtain on some harsh realities, making it clear that mental health isn't just something we talk about when it's convenient: it's something we need to talk about—loudly, openly, and without shame.

But we made it through.

In this chapter, we've looked at one of the most important questions: *Who's actually affected by trauma?* And the answer is clear—it's far more widespread than most people want to believe. Trauma isn't limited to those who've experienced combat, violent assaults, or natural disasters. It's not only about those with big, obvious traumas. It's affecting far more people than we like to admit—quietly shaping lives, relationships, and entire communities.

But there's another side to that question—another layer we haven't peeled back yet. Because sometimes, the person suffering isn't the one who lived through the trauma firsthand. Sometimes, it's the one who stood nearby. The one who tried to love them through it. The one who silently carried the emotional fallout. Because here's the truth most people miss: trauma is contagious. Not in the way a virus spreads through the air, but through proximity, connection, and emotional exposure. If you live close to someone who's struggling with unhealed trauma, it doesn't just stay contained—it seeps into your life, too. Slowly, quietly, sometimes without you even realizing it, until you're carrying symptoms of a pain you never personally experienced. That's what we're going to look at next. Because trauma doesn't just injure individuals—it ripples outward. And understanding that ripple is the key to healing not just survivors, but everyone trauma touches.

Let's talk about secondary PTSD.

CHAPTER 7

CONTAGIOUS SCARS

Jen Satterly spent years behind the camera, capturing the raw, gritty realities of the most elite warriors in the world. As the director of film and photography for a special operations training company, she was embedded with Navy SEALs, Green Berets, and Army Rangers, witnessing firsthand how these warriors pushed their bodies and minds to the brink in realistic, large-scale training missions designed to mimic the chaos of combat. But for Jen, it was more than just watching through a lens. She absorbed the weight of their stories, the brotherhood they shared, and the scars combat left behind—scars no camera could capture.

Jen wasn't just an observer. She felt the unspoken tension, the toll combat took on them even as they carried on with unshakable strength. The adrenaline-fueled missions, the long deployments, and the haunting memories stayed with them, and soon Jen would understand those same struggles on a deeply personal level. When she met Tom Satterly, she found herself standing at the front lines of a different battle.

Tom Satterly's life reads like something out of an action film, only it was all real. A Delta Force operator who spent twenty years in one of the military's most elite units, Tom lived through some of the most pivotal moments in modern warfare. His very first combat mission was the infamous Battle of Mogadishu, a grueling eighteen-hour firefight that became the longest since Vietnam, later immortalized in the film

Black Hawk Down. But that was only the beginning. Tom went on to lead missions that shaped America's military strategy.

As a soldier, Tom was the epitome of strength and resilience, earning five Bronze Star Medals (two with Valor). But like many war heroes, the battles didn't end when he left the battlefield. The shift from leading America's most dangerous missions to navigating civilian life was brutal. The intensity of combat, the adrenaline, the clear sense of purpose—it was all gone. And in its place were feelings of isolation, anger, and crushing depression. Tom had grown used to operating in an environment where showing weakness was a death sentence, and that mindset followed him home. The cocktail of pills, alcohol, and nightmares became Tom's new battlefield. His marriages failed one by one, and the emotional disconnect from his son only deepened.

But there was one bright spot amidst the chaos—Jen. She had met Tom while shooting a training exercise, and their connection quickly deepened beyond the professional realm. They started texting, calling, sharing their lives, and for the first time in years, Tom began to open up. He spoke about his failed marriages, the toll combat had taken on him, and the distance he felt from his son. Jen listened, and her presence became an anchor for Tom in ways neither of them had anticipated. However, as their relationship grew, so did Tom's inner demons. The burden of his trauma, combined with his fear of ruining yet another relationship, pushed him to the brink. The more he shoved those feelings down, the harder they fought back, until one day, sitting in his car with a pistol in his hand, Tom nearly ended it all.

As he sat there, contemplating how to pull the trigger, his phone buzzed. It was Jen. She was waiting for him at the bar with colleagues, unaware of just how bad the raging inside him had become. Her simple text—"Where are you? Are you okay?"—was enough to break the spell. The moment of finality slipped away as he put the gun down and went to meet her. That text saved Tom's life.

In the months that followed, Jen made it clear to Tom that he needed to get help. She had seen too many warriors like him suffer silently until it was too late, and she refused to let him be one of them. Jen gave Tom an ultimatum: seek therapy or lose her forever. Tom chose wisely: He chose to get help—and a life with Jen.

When Tom and Jen walked into my office, the resilience in their eyes was unmistakable—a strength born not just from enduring their own battles, but from standing together through them. I was struck by the depth of their bond, forged in the crucible of trauma and pain.

A conventional approach to PTSD/PTSI might have focused solely on Tom, as he exemplified everything we typically associate with trauma: combat, battles, and the haunting invisible wounds left by war. He was the decorated Delta Force veteran who had seen the worst of what humanity could offer. But the truth was, Tom wasn't the only one affected by trauma. Jen's story reveals a critical, often-overlooked reality—secondary PTSD/PTSI. This is the trauma experienced by those who love and live alongside someone suffering from PTSD/PTSI. As Tom's battles manifested in anger, isolation, and emotional withdrawal, those struggles seeped into Jen's life, pulling her from the role of observer into a personal war zone of her own.

What was once a partnership founded in love and support became a battlefield of emotional survival for Jen. She faced her own trauma, not from her own experiences of war, but from the fallout of Tom's unaddressed trauma. Her journey was not only about loving a man who had been through unimaginable experiences but about navigating the silent, insidious effects of secondary PTSD/PTSI.

Listening to Jen describe her struggles, I was reminded of my mother, who suffered silently under the weight of my father's trauma—a burden she bore until it claimed her life.

Jen's story and my own experiences with secondary PTSD/PTSI share some haunting parallels. Watching my mother live through the harsh realities of my father's untreated PTSD/PTSI taught me, early on, how trauma's reach can extend far beyond the person who experienced it firsthand. My father's trauma, born from wartime horrors in Cherkasy, cast an unshakeable shadow over our home. His unprocessed rage was like a slow poison, seeping into every corner of our lives and taking root in ways that none of us could escape.

My mother's story parallels Jen's in profound ways—both women became emotional fortresses for men shattered by combat trauma. As a physician, my mother approached suffering with clinical precision, yet her medical training offered no protection against the slow erosion of her own spirit.

In our austere household, where necessities barely outweighed wants, I witnessed the gradual dimming of a once-brilliant light. My father returned from war physically intact but carrying invisible wounds that bled into every aspect of our family life. My mother absorbed these wounds day after day, becoming both healer and casualty in an unwinnable battle. The stark simplicity of our home reflected the emotional restraint and emptiness that trauma so often leaves behind. There were no resources left for joy when survival consumed everything. My mother's face grew increasingly hollow, mirroring the internal emptying that occurs when one person carries another's unbearable pain. Secondary trauma isn't just sympathetic suffering: it's a contagion that spreads through intimate connection, claiming victims with the same ruthless efficiency as combat itself.

Her suicide came not as an abrupt rupture but as the final page of a long, agonizing chapter. The war had claimed her as surely as if she had served on its front lines. This understanding infuses my work with couples like Jen and Tom with both urgency and intimate knowledge. In their struggles, I recognize the same patterns that defined my childhood—the silent suffering, the gradual dissolution of identity, the desperate attempts to contain pain that refuses containment. My professional path emerged from this personal crucible, driven by the conviction that trauma's ripple effects through families can be interrupted before they claim more lives like my mother's.

Trauma is an invisible virus—it doesn't just harm the person at the center of the storm. It seeps outward, into the hearts and minds of everyone nearby, reshaping relationships and distorting the emotional landscape of entire families. Trauma silently infects those offering love and support, until they begin to carry symptoms that mirror the original wound. Those closest to trauma survivors often absorb the emotional weight: anxiety, sleeplessness, chronic unease. Some feel guilt, numbness, helplessness; others develop physical symptoms—tight muscles, chronic fatigue, lowered immunity. They haven't lived through the event itself, but they carry a version of it inside them just the same. Jen's story illustrates this. She was never deployed, never held a weapon, never heard the sound of mortar fire—but living beside Tom meant living inside his war. His trauma bled into her life.

I know this reality intimately. Growing up with a parent battling PTSD/PTSI, I learned early on that trauma doesn't confine itself to one person. It creates an emotional climate—one where others learn to tiptoe, to brace, to endure. Secondary trauma creeps in quietly. Loved ones may find themselves consumed by their partner's pain, losing focus, growing distant, or developing rigid thinking patterns. They may ride waves of sorrow, rage, or emotional numbness without knowing why. It's like living beside a fire: You don't have to be in the flames to feel the heat. Even at a distance, the smoke reaches you—filling your lungs, stinging your eyes, and staying long after the fire dies down. For those of us who've lived this truth, addressing secondary PTSD/PTSI isn't optional—it's essential. Because true healing isn't just about helping the primary survivor, it's about breaking the cycle. It's about recognizing trauma's ripple effect and stopping the spread before it claims another life, another mind, another heart.

My work today reaches beyond trauma survivors to those who support them. My mother's life—and her tragic end—taught me that trauma refuses to remain contained. It radiates outward, transforming family dynamics and burdening partners and children with a weight they neither understand or chose. This personal connection drives me to help couples like Jen and Tom who fight together despite overwhelming odds. Treating them wasn't about helping one individual, but healing two lives intertwined in the same battle from different fronts. Their willingness to face their pain together represented extraordinary courage—a couple who could have been destroyed by trauma but chose recovery instead.

Their story reinforces what I've always known: just as trauma spreads, so can healing. Supporting both survivors and their loved ones, untangling trauma's roots from family and community soil, has become my lifelong mission.

At this point, we've examined trauma's core nature and its impact beyond the brain to the entire body. We've uncovered how it traps people in the iron maiden of the mind, influencing everything from basic emotions to intimate relationships. Most importantly, we've seen how trauma refuses to exist in isolation, spreading like a virus through families, communities, and generations.

With these foundations established, we're ready to address the ultimate question: *If trauma is an injury, can we treat it? And if so, how?* Answering this has been my life's work—the point where my personal story, medical training, and commitment to healing finally converge. In the next chapter, we'll explore the science, breakthroughs, and methods that can break trauma's grip, redefining what healing makes possible.

CHAPTER 8

THE GOD SHOT

Let's press rewind a bit—back to 1984. Picture this: a young Eugene, starched white coat still crackling with newness, stethoscope slung around his neck like a badge of honor.

Fresh out of med school with textbook knowledge practically leaking from my ears, I was buzzing with the electric anticipation of following my father's scalpel-wielding footsteps. The surgical arena beckoned—that sterile battlefield where life and death tangoed under harsh lights, and I couldn't wait to join the dance.

Then life hurled not just a curveball, but a wrecking ball. When my mother's depression finally swallowed her whole and she took her life, leaving behind nothing but devastating questions, my carefully constructed medical identity shattered. The surgical resilience I'd been cultivating—that iron stomach and titanium nerves—dissolved like sutures in an infection. The OR's demanding rhythm, once thrilling, now felt like a jackhammer...I couldn't reconcile saving strangers while having failed to save the person who mattered most.

So, I wandered through medicine's corridors, trying doors that might lead somewhere less raw. Anesthesiology seemed promising—still adjacent to surgery's high-stakes world but buffered by machines and monitors.

Yet three months in, I felt like the perpetual benchwarmer watching the real players take the field—clipboard in hand, always analyzing the game but never feeling the rush of making the crucial play. Every day I'd suit up, warm up, but when the real medical drama kicked off, I was relegated to the sidelines. There I was, the once-promising surgeon, now essentially a pharmacological DJ, mixing sedative cocktails while the real medical drama unfolded on the other side of the sterile drape. The patient interaction had been reduced to a brief pre-op hello and a groggy post-op goodbye, with unconsciousness filling all the meaningful space between. I craved the messy, beautiful complexity of conscious human connection.

Then came pain medicine—a revelation wrapped in a specialty. Suddenly, I was tracing the topography of suffering with my fingertips, decoding the language of nerve and muscle. Each case was a mystery novel with somatic chapters, and I was both detective and healer.

For the first time since my mother's death, I felt the circuits reconnecting, the current of purpose flowing again. In pain medicine, I found more than a profession but a reconciliation—a way to transform my intimate knowledge of suffering into something that eased the burden for others.

In the early 2000s, a woman came into my office with neck pain so severe, it practically had its own gravitational pull. I took care of her neck pain using radiofrequency ablation, and, just when I thought we were done, she tossed out a side complaint: hot flashes. She'd tried every trick in the book, from hormone replacement to herbal remedies, and nothing worked. I spoke with my brother—a physician whose clinical judgment I deeply respected—and he suggested a procedure called the stellate ganglion block, or SGB.

I was intimately familiar with the procedure; I'd performed it regularly since the late '80s, during my residency at a VA hospital in Chicago. Back then, this nerve block was a standard treatment for severe hand pain, particularly for complex regional pain syndrome (CRPS), commonly called "burning arm syndrome." At the time, SGB was just one of many tools in my growing pain management toolkit. Little did I know, this simple nerve block would one day transform not only my career but my entire understanding of trauma. It would become the foundation for a breakthrough in treating something far more profound than just physical pain.

My brother's recommendation came as a surprise, but his reasoning was straightforward: SGB works to reduce excessive sweating in the extremities of CRPS patients, so perhaps it could help with her menopausal whole-body sweats. The sympathetic nervous system, after all, governs both localized and systemic sweating responses. I thought he might be grasping at straws—this was certainly an odd use of the procedure—but the physiological mechanism made enough sense to consider it. And given the patient's exhausted list of failed treatments, why not give it a "shot?" Sometimes the most revolutionary discoveries begin with a simple, "Well, it's worth trying."

My patient returned the next day, practically floating through the doorway, her face aglow with disbelief. "Doc, my hot flashes are GONE!" she announced, as if declaring she'd won the lottery.

I stood there, stethoscope frozen midair, thinking, "What in the world?" This was supposed to be a medical Hail Mary, not an actual solution. But the universe wasn't finished surprising me.

Around this time, I had a nurse—clinically brilliant but temperamentally...*challenging;* let's call her Anna. Premenopause, she'd been merely stern, the kind of no-nonsense professional who kept our office running with military precision. But when menopause hit, her personality transformed from sandpaper to shattered glass. The hallways practically crackled with tension when she approached. She'd erupt over misplaced charts or unanswered phones, her vocabulary suddenly rich with colorful expletives that would make a sailor blush, launched like verbal grenades at whoever stood in her path.

The office had become a minefield, with staff diving into supply closets to avoid her wrath. When prompted, she'd immediately blame the hot flashes—"You try thinking straight when you feel like you're being boiled alive from the inside out!" she'd snap, fanning herself furiously with whatever was in reach.

Finally, after a particularly volcanic day when several different staff members threatened to quit, I called her into my office. Half-serious, half-desperate, I laid it out: "ANNA, we have exactly two options here: either we try this nerve block that might—emphasis on might—help with your hot flashes, or I'm going to have to let you go. The choice is yours."

She glared at me with eyes that could have performed laser surgery, then nodded curtly. I suspect she was as exhausted by her own emotions as we were.

The next morning, I performed the stellate ganglion block, using the same technique I'd refined over years of treating CRPS patients. My reasoning was simple: if it could cool the inferno of her hot flashes, maybe—just maybe—it would take the edge off her temper too.

What happened next was nothing short of phenomenal. The transformation wasn't subtle or gradual—it was as if someone had flipped a switch. Within twenty-four hours, Hurricane Anna had dissipated into gentle spring showers. The woman who'd been launching verbal missiles was now the light of the break room. She spoke softly, listened patiently, and—most shocking of all—smiled. She actually smiled!

It was such a dramatic shift that the local newspaper ran a small piece about "medical mysteries," and someone from the office (anonymously, for obvious reasons) pinned it to our bulletin board, with a fluorescent-yellow highlighter circle around the paragraph about her "remarkable transformation."

I remember watching her calmly coach a new employee through a procedure, thinking, *those hot flashes must have been absolute torture,* but I didn't connect the deeper dots. The rest of the staff, meanwhile, whispered theories ranging from "secret therapy" to "personality transplant." I filed it away as a peculiar one-off, a medical footnote rather than a chapter opener.

Little did I know that those cases weren't anomalies: They were the first visible ripples of what would become a tidal wave of understanding about how trauma physically rewires not just the brain but the entire nervous system, and how a simple injection could sometimes reset what years of talk therapy couldn't touch.

About a year later, my original hot flash patient burst through my office door, her face flushed not with excitement this time, but with the unmistakable crimson glow of returning symptoms. "Doctor," she announced, dabbing perspiration from her hairline with a crumpled tissue, "the hot flashes are back." She'd just returned from a weeklong trip to Vegas, where apparently what happens in Vegas includes the resurrection of menopausal symptoms.

My jaw nearly hit the floor as the revelation struck. *Wait, what? It worked for an entire year?* The medical textbooks in my head frantically flipped pages—stellate ganglion blocks typically last a few months for pain conditions, not twelve. This wasn't just a fluke or coincidence; this was a pattern begging to be investigated. I reached for the phone before my patient had even left the office, punching in my brother's number with the urgency of someone who'd just discovered gold in their backyard.

"Send me more patients," I told him, not bothering with pleasantries. "Let's see if this actually works consistently." I could practically hear his eyebrows raising through the phone line.

Within weeks, they started arriving—a parade of women with identical stories but unique suffering. The results weren't just positive, they were transformative. Women who'd been existing rather than living were suddenly reclaiming their lives. Most heart-wrenching were the breast cancer survivors, warriors who'd fought the battle of their lives only to face a different kind of torture. They were required to take medications called aromatase inhibitors, like tamoxifen—lifesaving drugs that suppress estrogen and reduce cancer recurrence by about 35 percent. The cruel irony? These medications amplified menopausal symptoms to excruciating levels, turning occasional hot flashes into near-constant internal infernos.

I watched these women sitting in my waiting room, their clothes sticking to damp skin, portable fans whirring desperately in their hands, faces expressing a particular kind of exhaustion that comes from never getting relief. For them, life had become an impossible choice: endure round-the-clock misery or risk the cancer returning. The statistics were staggering—nearly half abandoned their critical medication within the first six months. Imagine the desperation that drives someone to stop taking a drug designed to keep deadly cancer at bay.

"It feels like I'm being cooked from the inside out, all day, every day," one woman told me, her eyes rimmed red from fatigue. "I'd rather face whatever comes than live like this for five more years."

Another described how she'd stand in front of her open refrigerator at 3 a.m., pressing frozen vegetables against her chest, neck, anywhere that might cool the internal furnace, knowing all along she was gambling with her life by discontinuing her medication.

Hot flashes, night sweats, insomnia, and a libido nosedive weren't just symptoms—they were wrecking balls demolishing these women's lives from the inside out. One patient confided in me, her voice barely above a whisper, "My husband says sleeping next to me is like cuddling with a cold, wet fish." She laughed, but the pain in her eyes told a different story. Another described how she'd changed her bedsheets three times in a single night, each time peeling away linens so drenched you could wring them out like laundry on washday.

These women weren't just tired—they were bone-weary, soul-exhausted. Then came the stellate ganglion block—a procedure so seemingly simple it was almost anticlimactic. A thin needle, guided by ultrasound, delivering targeted relief to a tiny cluster of nerves. The transformation that followed, however, was anything but simple. Women who'd shuffled into my office, shoulders hunched under the weight of their misery, would bounce back for follow-ups with the energy of someone who'd discovered a fountain of youth.

In 2005, the *Chicago Tribune* got wind of the work I was doing and reached out for a story. I was hopeful this would be the moment to spread the word, making this relief accessible to so many more women. So, I opened my doors, ready to share every detail about the breakthroughs happening right there in Chicago. But when the article hit the stands, my stomach dropped as soon as I read the opening line. *Uh-oh.* This wasn't going to be the celebration I'd imagined.

They opened with a shocker: *"Bianca Kennard, a beautiful 35-year-old breast cancer survivor, was so desperate to get rid of her hot flashes, she let Dr. Lipov plunge a three-inch needle into her neck."* And with that, they branded me: "the needle plunger."

It didn't stop there. They went straight to the heads of major institutions—Northwestern University and Rush University, where I'd trained—and every one of them threw me under the bus. They dismissed the procedure, calling it everything from reckless to experimental. Their verdict was essentially, "Sure, it works—but he doesn't know *why* it works." They dismissed it as medical heresy.

The *Tribune* article sparked something fierce in me: I wasn't about to sit around and let anyone call my work a fluke. I was determined to dig into the science behind the stellate ganglion block and prove this treatment was more than a shot in the dark. So, I threw myself into research, combing through every medical journal I could get my hands on, hunting for clues to understand why this nerve block was working the way it was.

I dove into a mountain of research, reading over 3,000 publications dissecting each one for insights that could help me understand exactly *why* the stellate ganglion block worked the way it did. I was on a mission to connect the dots—and I wasn't stopping until I had the answers. After wading through stacks of studies, one particular paper from Finland caught my attention. It was on a procedure called T2 sympathetic clipping—a highly invasive operation involving two large tubes inserted into the chest to reach the T2 ganglia, often done to treat excessive hand sweating. But here's where things got intriguing: tucked away in the study was an observation that patients who had undergone T2 clipping reported a surprising reduction in PTSD symptoms.

PTSD relief? From a nerve block? I was floored. Here I was, researching sweating treatments, and suddenly I stumbled onto a much larger discovery. My mind was racing; what was the connection here?

From there, I started digging even deeper, pulling apart the anatomy and neurobiology to understand the connection.

I found that the T2 ganglia in the chest sent nerve signals up to the stellate ganglion in the neck, which then relayed those signals to the brain's emotional center. It was like finding a direct pathway to the brain's trauma circuitry, a doorway into the part of the brain that keeps us locked in "danger mode." This was a breakthrough. It wasn't just some accidental effect—the nerve pathways were all connected. Boom.

That was a lightbulb moment: if T2 sympathetic clipping could reduce PTSD symptoms, the simpler, less invasive stellate ganglion block could potentially do the same, without the high risks.

T2 clipping, after all, was a grueling procedure, involving tubes the size of an index finger being inserted into a patient's chest, pushing the lung aside—a complex and risky ordeal. But the stellate ganglion block? It was safe, took ten to fifteen minutes, and, theoretically, it could yield similar results. I had to test this theory. My mission had taken on a new urgency. The stakes had just gone from a sweating cure to a potential breakthrough in PTSD treatment.

The next step was clear: it was time to see if the stellate ganglion block could offer real relief for those suffering from PTSD.

My first patient was a man who had been brutally attacked in a robbery. In the months since, he'd been on a downward spiral, haunted by flashbacks and terror, barely holding on. By the time he found his way to my office, he was a ghost wearing human skin. His eyes—perpetually ringed with the charcoal smudges of sleeplessness—darted around my waiting room like a cornered animal's. His last stop before a psychiatric ward was my operating room.

I performed the stellate ganglion block. What happened next still stops me in my tracks when I think about it. Within ten minutes—*ten minutes*—his breathing deepened. His shoulders dropped away from his ears. And then, like watching a time-lapse video of ice melting, his face changed. The tension lines around his mouth softened. His jaw unclenched. And those haunted eyes—those eyes that had seen horrors replaying on endless loop—they cleared. Focused. Saw the present instead of the past.

"It's quiet," he said, wonder breaking his voice. "My head...it's finally quiet."

I just stood there smiling, trying to process what I was witnessing. He'd tried conventional treatments—the best modern psychiatry had to offer—but they'd barely made a dent in his suffering. Yet in less time than it takes to watch a sitcom, something fundamental had shifted. It wasn't just symptom relief—it was like watching someone step back into their own skin, reclaim their own existence.

In the months that followed, his transformation held. The flashbacks that had ambushed him dozens of times daily became rare visitors. The hypervigilance that had kept him perpetually exhausted loosened its grip. He started sleeping through the night, reconnecting with friends, even planning for a future he'd previously been unable to imagine existing long enough to see.

"I don't understand it," he told me during a follow-up visit, a man resurrected, "but I'm not questioning it either. You gave me my life back."

What I couldn't tell him was that he had given me something, too—a glimpse into a treatment possibility that would transform not only my medical practice but my understanding of how deeply the body holds trauma, and how directly we might be able to release it. This was the turning point, the moment when I knew this was bigger than I could have imagined. My research was no longer a quest for validation; it was a mission to bring life-changing relief to as many people as possible. One patient led to another, and soon enough, the impact of the procedure began to ripple outward.

Veterans like Jason Brown, a Special Forces soldier who had lived through unspeakable horrors, found hope where there had been none. Jason had been haunted by his experiences overseas, struggling to survive in the aftermath. After the procedure, he looked at me with a quiet clarity and said, "Before, I felt like I was going one hundred miles per hour all the time. After the SGB, I'm down to twenty." We'd just managed to release the gas pedal, and in that instant, his whole life transformed before my eyes.

With each patient who walked out of my office straighter, lighter, somehow more present than when they'd entered, that fire in my gut burned hotter. I'd lie awake at night, staring at ceiling shadows, my mind racing with visions of the millions still suffering—men and women standing at the edges of bridges, children curled into tight balls of fear in their beds, families fractured by the invisible walls trauma builds between people who love each other.

And always, *always,* my mother's face would float into these midnight reflections. I'd imagine her sitting in my treatment room, that perpetual tension in her shoulders finally easing as the treatment took effect. I'd visualize the moment when her eyes—so much like mine—would clear of that haunted look they'd carried for as long as I could remember. *What if this had been around for her? What if, instead of a rope and a chair, she'd had access to this shot of hope?* The weight of that question was sometimes crushing, but it was also fuel, propelling me forward with the force of all that unresolved grief. Every time a patient tells me, *"I finally feel like myself again,"* I feel her. I feel her hand on my back, steady and familiar, as if to say I've managed to turn something terrible into something good. In those moments, I can almost hear her whisper, *"Well done."* It's not enough to bring her back into my life—and it never will be. But maybe, just maybe, I've saved a child from living with the absence of a mother or father. Maybe I've helped someone stay who would have otherwise left.

Data piled up like autumn leaves—case after case showing dramatic reductions in symptoms that had resisted every other intervention. Eventually, my work gained traction, attracting the attention of a Chicago lobbyist who saw the potential and helped us secure letters of support from key leaders, including then-Senator Obama. This was no longer just about helping individuals—it was becoming a movement, a chance to rewrite the rules on trauma and give countless people a second shot at life.

And then came another breakthrough.

In 2012, a young Marine sniper walked into my office—a man honed in discipline and toughness. But as he took a seat, I could see that he was a man on the edge, sitting in my office with his wife, both of them broken and tear-streaked, and he was looking at me with the hollow eyes of someone who'd lost hope. He was clear: "Doc, I'm going to kill myself."

I suggested the hospital, but he dismissed the idea with such visceral revulsion you'd think I'd recommended he bathe in acid. His whole body recoiled, shoulders hunching as if to make himself a smaller target.

"No hospitals," he rasped, eyes darting toward the exit. "They'll lock me up and throw away the key." For him, the hospital wasn't a place of healing—it was a cage with fluorescent lighting, a trap baited with promises of help that would snap shut and steal what little freedom he had left. The tremor in his hands intensified, his knuckles bleaching white as he gripped the edge of his chair.

"Just give me the shot," he pleaded, voice cracking like thin ice underfoot. "The shot is the only thing I'm asking for. Nothing else." His eyes—bloodshot and haunted—locked onto mine with the desperate intensity of a drowning man spotting a life preserver. I knew exactly what he wanted: a stellate ganglion block, the procedure that had helped others crawl back from trauma's edge.

But this was uncharted territory. My other patients had been struggling, yes, but stable. This man was balanced on a knife's edge of despair so sharp I could almost see him bleeding out emotionally right there in my office.

In that moment, the weight of the Hippocratic oath felt like an anvil on my chest: "First, do no harm." But what was the greater harm here? Performing an unorthodox treatment for severe psychiatric distress? Or turning away someone who had summoned every last ounce of courage to ask for help, knowing he would seek no other? My mother's face flashed before me—her eyes carrying that same bottomless desperation in the weeks before she took her life. I remembered how the system had failed her, how the textbook approaches had left her feeling more isolated, more hopeless. How she'd reached out in her own way, and no one had recognized the depth of her pain until it was too late.

"Doctor," his voice cut through my memories, his gaze unwavering despite the tears now streaming unchecked down his face. "I'm not going anywhere else after this. You understand what I'm saying?" The implication hung in the air between us, heavy and undeniable. This wasn't just his last stop for medical help—it might be his last stop, period.

Medical school had prepared me for many things—calculating medication dosages, diagnosing rare conditions, delivering devastating news—but not for this moment where textbook ethics collided with raw human suffering. There was no algorithm, no clinical pathway to follow. Just a man in anguish and a doctor with the theoretical ability to ease it, separated by a chasm of professional guidelines and uncertainty.

I looked down at his intake form, at the shaky signature that had trailed off the line as if even writing his name required more strength than he possessed. Then I looked back at his face—a battlefield map of pain, fear, and a flickering, fading hope that I might be different from all the others who had failed him. My decision crystallized like frost on a winter window. Sometimes medicine isn't about following maps—it's about making them.

"Come back tomorrow morning," I said quietly. "We'll do the block."

The relief that washed over his features was like watching someone surface after being underwater too long—desperate, grateful, reborn. I spent that night wrestling with the voices of every cautious medical professor who had ever warned against improvisation. But louder than all of them was my mother's voice, and the silence that had followed when that voice was gone.

The next day, with steady hands that belied my churning thoughts, I did the block—targeting C6, the standard spot in the neck's stellate ganglion. When he came out, I looked into his eyes, hoping for a spark of change, but he looked at me and said, "I'm still going to kill myself."

The words slammed into me like a physical blow, shattering any fragile hope I'd been harboring. It felt like the air had been sucked out of the room, leaving nothing but a vacuum of despair. This was it—the last line of defense, and it hadn't worked.

Then, lightning struck my memory—my experience in Norway, where I had tried a higher-level block located in the C3 ganglion. Same procedure, slightly different location. Maybe his block hadn't been effective because of the location. There were no guarantees, no research papers I could cite supporting this approach specifically for PTSD.

My medical training flickered through my mind like warning lights on a dashboard. Should I give it a try? The question pounded in my skull with each heartbeat. I felt backed into a corner, torn between two impossible choices, the weight of his life pressing down on my shoulders until I could barely breathe. My training screamed caution—there was no guarantee it would work, and if it went wrong, the consequences would rest squarely on my conscience. But then there was the man sitting in front of me, his eyes as vacant as abandoned buildings, his voice echoing with the hollow timbre of someone who had already begun to disconnect from this world.

I explained the alternative procedure in meticulous detail—the location, the risks, the complete absence of clinical precedent for this specific application. I prompted him again, practically begged him, to seek out psychiatric help. But he was granite in his resolve, unmovable as a mountain. His gaze locked with mine, unflinching.

"You're my last shot, Doc. There's no plan B here."

His wife stood beside him, her face contorted and swollen with tears that had carved salty rivulets down her cheeks. When our eyes met, hers confirmed what I already knew—he meant every word. If I refused, she would be planning a funeral instead of a recovery. How could I say no? The question thundered in my ears. How could I let him walk away without trying everything—absolutely everything—within my power? My heart was a lead weight in my chest, pulled down by the burden of his plea and the ghostly whispers of my own past failures. Cold sweat beaded on my brow, each droplet a testament to the magnitude of this moment.

With equal parts hope and terror churning in my gut like oil and water, I took him back into the operating room. My fingers moved with the precision born from thousands of procedures, but my thoughts were a hurricane of doubt and determination. *What if this was the wrong choice? What if I'm making it worse?* But his desperate pleas echoed in my mind, drowning out the doubts. This was a man begging not for comfort but for existence itself.

The silence in the room was suffocating as I prepared the injection for the C3 ganglion. As I inserted the needle, guided by X-ray to that precise point on his neck, time seemed to stretch and distort. Each second became an eternity, every millimeter of movement magnified a hundredfold. My senses heightened to almost painful acuity—the slight resistance as the needle penetrated tissue, the sound of his shallow, nervous breathing, the antiseptic smell that suddenly seemed overwhelming in its chemical potency. His life—and perhaps the future of trauma treatment—teetered on the edge of this moment, not knowing if we were about to plummet or soar.

When the procedure ended, we waited in that suspended animation that follows moments of great consequence. The tension was palpable, thick enough to require a scalpel to slice through. I watched his face with the intensity of a scientist monitoring a once-in-a-lifetime experiment, searching for any sign—a twitch of an eyelid, a flicker of emotion across his features—anything that might telegraph success or failure. My own breath caught in my chest, afraid that even the slightest exhalation might tip the scales one way or another.

Then, slowly, he opened his eyes. He looked at me, and for a moment, I saw something different—a glimmer, a subtle shift like the first silver edge of dawn breaking through night. He raised his hand, palm open. I raised mine to meet it, and the sound of our high five cracked through the silence like thunder after lightning.

"I'm good, Doc," he said, his lips curling into a small but genuine smile that reached his eyes—eyes that now held a spark of life that had been extinguished minutes before.

I stood there, rooted to the spot, trying to process what had just happened. Relief crashed over me like a tsunami, mingled with disbelief that threatened to sweep me away. *Had we really just done it? Had I found a way to manually "reset" his fight-or-flight response with nothing but a needle and a theory?* I watched him walk out of my office that day, his shoulders no longer bearing the invisible weight that had bent him almost to breaking, his steps lighter, as if gravity itself had lessened its hold.

And the most incredible thing—it lasted. In the years following the treatment, he had no return of the extreme PTSD symptoms that had nearly driven him to end his life. No flashbacks that hijacked his consciousness. No paralyzing anxiety that imprisoned him in his own home. No nights spent pacing until dawn broke the darkness. It wasn't just a fleeting moment of hope, a temporary reprieve from suffering. It was real. It was transformative. It worked. And in that realization, everything I thought I knew about trauma treatment tilted on its axis, opening a door I hadn't even known existed.

In the months that followed that incident, I dove into further research to understand why the second procedure had worked when the first hadn't. This wasn't just luck; I knew that much. I had to understand what made this dual-block approach effective. So, I plunged into research, and began combing through countless studies, looking for anything that could shed light on the nerve pathways. That's when I found a book published in 1956 by James Moore, out of print since 1972. Hidden within its pages was a diagram—an anatomical map that showed the exact pathways the sympathetic nerves followed. Half the nerves, it turned out, traveled up through C6 to the brain, while the other half followed a higher route up to the superior cervical ganglion at C3. The two pathways connected to separate parts of the brain, meaning that by targeting both points, we were effectively covering more ground.

I had stumbled upon something monumental: a way to reach the brain's core threat response centers through what we would come to call the Dual Sympathetic Reset (DSR). And it wasn't just a theory—it was a treatment that could potentially change the lives of trauma survivors around the world.

The gravity of that day hit me fully. I wasn't just a doctor treating pain anymore. I was standing at the edge of a breakthrough that could bring peace to thousands, if not more. And as I thought of my mother, I knew that no matter the challenges ahead, I would do everything in my power to make this treatment available to anyone who needed it.

The stellate ganglion block was more than a medical breakthrough: It was a lifeline for those who'd been left to navigate trauma's unyielding grip with nothing more than coping mechanisms. Finally, there was a way to reach into the brain's darkest corners and flip the switch—bringing the mind out of survival mode and back to a place of calm. And for me, every patient I helped was one step closer to honoring my mother's legacy and changing the landscape of trauma treatment forever.

Since the discovery of using the stellate ganglion block to treat PTSD/PTSI, and further developing the breakthrough Dual Sympathetic Reset procedure, I've had the opportunity to testify on PTSD treatment before the US House Committee on Veterans' Affairs in 2010. In collaboration with neuroscientists, I've established myself as the world's leading authority on the physiology of PTSD. I've been honored to have my work published in top medical journals such as *Biological Psychiatry, Current Psychiatry, Military Medicine, Pain Research & Treatment, Psychiatric Annals,* the *Journal of Anesthesia & Clinical Research,* the *Journal of Trauma and Treatment, The Lancet,* and *Pain Practice.* Beyond the academic circles, my research was featured in *The Wall Street Journal,* the *Los Angeles Times,* the *Chicago Tribune, USA Today, Wired, Playboy, Univision,* and *Stars and Stripes.* I've also shared my insights on ABC, NBC, and WGN. (By the way, it was the article published in *Playboy* that coined the term *"The God Shot"*—and it stuck.)

But for me, it's never been about the publications or the media coverage—it's about the people whose lives have been changed. I've had the immense privilege of treating thousands of remarkable individuals (and even dogs!)—like Michael, Katie, Max, and Trevor. People like Tom and Jen Satterly, who have faced experiences that most could never imagine. Each of them came to me carrying the invisible weight of trauma, a burden that had grown unbearable.

When Tom and Jen Satterly came to my office, they were both weighed down by Tom's combat trauma and the toll it had taken on their relationship. The SGB procedure became a game changer for both of them.

Hearing Jen recount her experience was profoundly moving. She shared, "I was awake, looking at Tom laying on a patient bed in the next room. He'd been put under anesthesia. Then Dr. Lipov put the shot in my neck—it wasn't pleasant, but it wasn't terrible and only lasted for about thirty seconds. Afterward, he bent over me, asked how I felt, and I can't really explain—it was a mix of euphoria, relief, sadness, and joy all at the same time. Tears started pouring out of me. He rested his forehead on mine and said, *'I know, I know,'* which only made me cry harder."

Laying there, Jen felt lighter. Something significant was missing—she realized that the constant sense of waiting for conflict or confrontation was gone. "After thirty minutes of sobbing, I laughed and told Dr. Lipov that he broke me. He said, 'Welcome to repressed emotional experience.' I think he was emotional, too, and told me he wished his mom and dad could have had the shot—that they might still be here."

Two weeks after the procedure, Jen was feeling empowered in ways she hadn't imagined. She no longer walked on eggshells, fearful of setting Tom off. She found herself singing in her car again, putting the top down, music blasting, feeling freer than she had since high school. It was a joyful, carefree feeling she hadn't experienced since before the traumas of her past. She noticed that old insecurities and fears seemed to fade away—like her hesitance to eat in front of others. She recalled, "Tom and I were at a huge group buffet. I was starving and went first, filled up my plate with everyone watching, and I didn't even notice until Tom said something." She felt less timid, less afraid, and she was no longer a pushover.

Tom's experience was also memorable for everyone who was in the room on the day of his treatment. Coming out of twilight anesthesia, before fully conscious, a part of Tom's mind processed the medical setting and concluded that he had been captured. He began thrashing against the restraints, shouting, "I'm going to kill every motherf--ker in this room!" But then, he saw Jen. The sight of her snapped him out of the delusion, and his demeanor immediately softened.

A few minutes after the injections, Tom began to notice something he couldn't remember ever feeling—calm. "I realized this heavy blanket of worry, the feeling that I'm late for something or something's wrong...it was gone. I felt happy. I wasn't agitated. I could breathe—*really* breathe." Visual proof was evident in his pre- and post-scans, showing remarkable changes.

Jen would later recount a moment during their walk in Chicago when a man startled them. Tom, rather than reacting with rage or hypervigilance, simply said, "Step back, don't startle people." She knew instantly that a week earlier, the encounter would have gone very differently.

Tom found he could do things out of routine, without the anxiety that had once gripped him. He could be in crowded rooms without feeling overwhelmed by anger or hypervigilance. He could sleep through the night, wake up with a positive outlook instead of dread. And perhaps the most important change for both of them—he could now take a beat before reacting. He had found a sense of peace that had eluded him for years.

Tom's perspective has remained hopeful: "I've been happier than I've ever been. Now I know I can function like a normal human being. The stories I've heard from other warriors after SGB or DSR have been remarkable—they can hold down jobs, they can get on planes. This is life-changing."

Michael, Katie, Max, Trevor, and the Satterlys all found their paths to healing through this treatment. Each story is different, but the common theme is undeniable: it is possible to break free from the invisible chains of trauma. The stellate ganglion block isn't just about suppressing symptoms—it's about giving people back their lives, their joy, their peace. Every one of them found something they thought they had lost forever—hope.

For Michael, recovery meant finally being able to sleep—full, uninterrupted nights of rest that gave him the energy to face each day without the dark cloud of exhaustion looming over him. It meant stepping out from the shadows of constant hypervigilance, no longer feeling the need to look over his shoulder at every moment. With the grip of trauma loosening, Michael was finally able to focus on school. The fog that had once kept him from understanding lessons began to lift, allowing him to concentrate, absorb information, and even enjoy learning. His teachers saw a change—a boy who once struggled just to sit still was now engaging, asking questions, and making progress. The fear and tension that had dominated his life for so long started to fade, replaced by curiosity and a sense of belonging he had never known before. For Michael, recovery was more than just surviving—it was about finally being able to thrive, to learn, and to hope for a future beyond trauma.

For Katie, the treatment meant rediscovering her emotions—seeing colors more vividly, feeling joy in the little things, and opening herself up to genuine connections that she had long thought were beyond her reach. It allowed her to relax, to feel alive without the specter of fear lurking at every corner, and to experience touch and intimacy without the nausea of past trauma.

For Max, recovery meant shedding the street-worn armor he'd built just to survive. The snarling, hyperalert posture that once kept everyone at bay began to soften. With time, the constant tension in his body gave way to something unfamiliar—ease. As his nervous system calmed, so did his spirit. He stopped scanning for threats and started looking to Emily—not only with obedience but with trust. Day by day, Max found his way back to himself—more than the tough survivor, but the dog he was always meant to be: loyal, steady, and finally safe.

For Trevor, recovery meant finally being able to exhale. The tightness in his chest that had been there for so many years loosened, allowing him to breathe deeply without the weight of the past crushing him. The grip of traumatic memories finally loosened, giving Trevor not just hope for the future, but also the strength to genuinely reconnect with his family, particularly his children. For the first time in years, those moments of connection felt authentic, not overshadowed by an undercurrent of anxiety. Though Trevor continued with therapy to address the deeper layers of his trauma, the difference was palpable—with his nervous system no longer in a constant state of fight or flight, real progress became possible.

For David Allen, the treatment was nothing short of life-changing. Before, he lived in a constant state of overdrive—snapping at his kids for minor things, shutting down emotionally with his wife, reacting to the world like it was always on fire. But after the treatment, something shifted. The noise quieted. The space between stimulus and response widened, giving him room to breathe, to think, to choose. He could sit at the dinner table and actually enjoy the sound of his kids' laughter instead of flinching at every sudden movement. He could look his wife in the eyes without the weight of guilt and distance. For the first time in years, David wasn't just surviving—he was living.

A few weeks after treating a first responder and his wife, my office phone lit up with his number. Not unusual—follow-up calls were routine—but something about this one felt different from the moment I answered.

"Doc," he said, his voice cracking like ice in warm whiskey, swimming with an emotion I couldn't immediately place. "I've got good news."

I leaned back in my chair, smiling into the receiver with the kind of automatic response you develop after years of practice. "Well, congratulations!" I offered, assuming he was calling about symptom improvement or perhaps returning to work—the usual victories we celebrated.

"No," he interrupted, his voice suddenly urgent, almost reverent. "You don't get it. We traced it back—we conceived the same day I got the SGB. That was the day *everything* changed."

The pen I'd been fidgeting with froze between my fingers. For years, they'd battled infertility with the same grim determination they'd brought to fighting his PTSD. Something shifted that day, something more profound than even I had understood. When his nervous system calmed—when that perpetual storm of adrenaline and cortisol finally abated—his body remembered how to do more than just survive: It remembered how to create life.

I sat there, stunned into silence, watching sunlight dance through my office window. In all my research, all my clinical planning, all my hopes for what the SGB could accomplish, I'd never anticipated this. We'd focused on symptoms—the hypervigilance, the insomnia, the flashbacks—not on the ripple effects that might spread when those symptoms subsided.

"Doc? You still there?" he prompted.

"I'm here," I managed, swallowing. "I'm just...that's incredible news."

"It's because of you," he said simply. "Before the shot, I was...I wasn't really there, you know? Even when I was physically present. It was like I was watching my life from behind bulletproof glass. But after...it was like someone washed the glass clean, then removed it entirely. I could feel again. I could connect. I could be *present.*"

As I hung up the phone, I stared at my calendar of upcoming patients, suddenly seeing each name not only as an individual suffering, but as the center of a constellation—connected to partners, children, friends, colleagues. Each treatment potentially restoring not just one life, but the intricate web of relationships surrounding it. And just like that, we had our very first SGB baby—a miracle I'd never thought to include in my research data, yet perhaps the most profound outcome of all. A new life, conceived through the union of two people and through the restoration of a nervous system that had finally remembered how to live rather than merely survive.

Over time, the results spoke for themselves—an efficacy rate of 80 to 85 percent, and with barely any side effects. The stellate ganglion block (SGB), especially when combined with the Dual Sympathetic Reset (DSR), became a force to be reckoned with. Against conventional treatments, it stood unmatched—and when paired with psychotherapy, it turned into a powerhouse. Precision guided by ultrasound, the procedure took just ten to twenty minutes, but those few minutes carried the potential to deliver instant, life-altering change.

The stories I've shared with you here are just a handful out of the hundreds—warriors, first responders, survivors of all kinds—who walked in carrying the weight of a nervous system stuck in overdrive and walked out with a shot at reclaiming their life. We've answered one of the biggest questions: *Can trauma actually be healed, or are we just supposed to cope forever?* It's clear now—true healing is possible. Not someday. Not in theory. Right now.

So that brings us to the next question—the one the skeptics and the curious alike always ask: *How does this actually work?* What's happening under the surface? Is this just a placebo effect—or is there something measurable, something biological, something real happening inside the body? That's exactly where we're headed next.

CHAPTER 9

THIS ISN'T WOO-WOO—IT'S SCIENCE

Science has always been my love language. Not the sterile, jargon-filled textbook kind, but the kind that solves real-world problems. The kind that looks at something seemingly impossible and says, "Watch me."

When I first started exploring this breakthrough in trauma treatment, I was met with more eye rolls than enthusiastic nods. Colleagues would lean back, arms crossed, wearing that classic skeptical smirk that screams, "Here we go again. Another maverick with another miracle cure."

I get it: I've been that skeptical doctor myself more times than I can count. But here's the thing about science: it doesn't care about your skepticism. It doesn't bow to tradition or popularity. Science is ruthlessly objective. It demands proof. Cold, hard, measurable evidence. So when I tell you that we've discovered a way to actually reset the trauma response in the body—not manage it, not cope with it, but fundamentally change it—I'm not asking you to believe me. I'm inviting you to look at the evidence. To examine the data. To see for yourself.

This chapter isn't about selling you a dream. It's about breaking down exactly what happens when we treat trauma as the physiological injury it truly is. We're going to get technical and a little "science-y," but I promise—I'll keep it as far from medical mumbo jumbo as possible. Think of this as a backstage pass to how the human body really works when trauma takes hold, and how we can finally—truly—help it heal. So, let's break it down simply, piece by piece. Let's start with the first question: *How does the procedure actually work?*

You remember that car engine analogy from earlier? Good. Because I want you to picture your body as a high-performance machine. When danger hits, your system slams the gas pedal—hard. That's your sympathetic nervous system firing up. Fight-or-flight mode. You're built to handle short bursts of emergency—running from a predator, escaping a burning building, dodging an oncoming threat. It's primal. It works. In a healthy system, once the danger is over, the engine slows. You downshift. Coast. The heart rate comes down. The body finds rhythm again. The threat's gone. You're safe now.

The problem? Trauma doesn't know when to let off the gas. That gas pedal stays jammed to the floor. And it stays there. Your amygdala—your internal alarm system—gets stuck in high alert, scanning every room, every face, every silence for danger that might not even be there. And you stop being the driver. The sympathetic nervous system hijacks the wheel, and suddenly your body is speeding full tilt through life with no brakes. You're just along for the ride, gripping the edges, praying you don't spin out. It's not subtle. You feel it everywhere. You're swerving through conversations like they're minefields. Snapping without knowing why. Lying awake at 3 a.m., like someone's coming for you, even when the room is still. Your digestion is wrecked. Your heart's racing. Your sex drive has vanished. You're exhausted and wired at the same time. You can practically hear the metal groaning under the pressure, smell the burn in your nervous system. Everything in you is screaming for a red light—a moment to breathe. But there isn't one. *Not unless you interrupt the loop.* And most of the time, the brakes people reach for to try and stop that revved up engine are drugs—because in a system stuck on overdrive, medication often becomes the only available brake.

That's where the stellate ganglion block comes in. It doesn't just soothe the symptoms. It goes straight to the stuck pedal—the signal loop between your body and brain—and gives it a hard reset. It's like popping the hood, cutting the feedback loop between your brain's panic button and your body's reaction, and letting the engine cool down. For the first time in years, maybe decades, the system stops flooring it. And for many people, the moment it happens, you can feel it—like someone just lifted their foot off the gas. And for the first time in a long time... you can breathe

The longer you stay in this max-alert, high-speed state, the more you get trapped in this Danger Loop. It's like being locked into a state of red alert, where every corner seems to hide an invisible enemy, even if, logically, you know there's nothing there. Your brain just can't turn it off. The amygdala—your internal siren—is caught in a loop, constantly blaring "Danger! Danger!" like the Robot from *Lost in Space.* Only, you're not in space, and there's no real enemy in sight. Just an unending sense that something bad is always about to happen.

As we've seen in the stories of Michael, Katie, Max, Trevor, and the Satterlys, this relentless high alert mode drains you completely, siphoning your mental and physical reserves like gas leaking from a punctured tank. You're left utterly exhausted but unable to rest. You're surrounded by people, but unable to truly connect. Even during the moments that should be calm, you're bracing for impact, waiting for that next disaster that never comes. Trauma becomes a thief, robbing you of the ability to relax, to feel safe, to just let go. It's a vicious cycle—one that the brain can't simply "snap out of" on its own.

When you start to feel yourself spinning out of control—sleepless nights, constant tension, feeling like you're bracing for impact every minute—you might decide it's time to reach out for help.

Standard treatment usually means medication, maybe mixed with talk therapy. And sure, for a while, it feels like the car is starting to stabilize: The chaos eases up and you're not spinning out as wildly.

But then come the side effects—your mind doesn't feel as sharp, there's a bit of a lag, some weird "noise" in the system. Maybe your emotions don't respond the way they used to, or you're not running on all cylinders anymore. But hey, at least you're not totally out of control, right?

But here's the catch: medication doesn't release that gas pedal. No, that's still pressed down, hard. Medication has just helped you push the emergency brake, so now you're driving with one foot on the brake and the other still glued to the gas pedal. The sympathetic nervous system, the part of you responsible for fight-or-flight, is still revving like an engine stuck on full throttle. You're holding it back, but only by sheer force.

So, you've got the brake and the gas pedal both pressed. Medications help keep the car from going totally nuts, but underneath, the engine is straining, trying to break free. Your body is working overtime to contain that pent-up energy, but the moment you lift your foot off the brake, the whole system risks spinning out again.

Talk therapy can be incredibly valuable. It gives you space to speak the unspeakable, to be seen and heard, to finally put words to what's been buried deep in your nervous system. That kind of safety matters. There's undeniable relief in being able to say, *This happened...*, and to have someone say, *You're not crazy for how it changed you.*

But here's the problem: if your nervous system is still stuck in survival mode, talk therapy alone can feel like stepping on the gas when all you need is a brake.

Every time you dive into those memories—no matter how skilled the therapist, no matter how safe the room—you're dragging your body right back into the battlefield. You're reactivating the alarm system without first disarming the bomb. And that means every aha moment comes at a cost: more emotional flooding, more physiological exhaustion, more spinning your wheels in a system already running on fumes.

Enter the stellate ganglion block.

When we inject a local anesthetic near this small but mighty bundle of nerves, two critical things happen. First, norepinephrine levels drop like a rock—usually within the first ten to fifteen minutes. It's like flipping a circuit breaker in a house that's been dangerously overloaded. That constant electrical surge—the flood of stress chemicals keeping your system on edge—gets cut off. The gas pedal finally lifts. And just like that, the body gets a chance to downshift, to breathe.

For about 60 percent of patients, that one moment brings immediate, marked relief. But here's the real magic—what happens underneath the surface, beyond the numbing and the quieting of the storm. As we touched on in a previous chapter, severe trauma doesn't just flood your system with norepinephrine. It also releases something called nerve growth factor (NGF)—a substance that tells your sympathetic nerves to sprout new branches. Imagine a tree growing wild, limbs reaching in all directions. These branches aren't helpful—they're hyperreactive pathways, making it even easier for your system to stay in fight-or-flight. Each new branch is like a fresh antenna tuned to danger. They don't just grow—they release more norepinephrine, amplifying the signal and reinforcing the trauma loop. Your body, in an attempt to survive, literally rewires itself to stay stuck. The gas pedal isn't just pressed down—it's bolted to the floor.

Now here's where the SGB changes everything. The anesthetic doesn't just cut off the norepinephrine surge—it also lowers NGF levels, which are required to keep those extra nerve branches alive. And when NGF drops, something beautiful happens: the branches begin to wither. The overgrowth prunes itself. You go from ten overactive, trauma-wired nerves to five. From a screaming emergency broadcast to something closer to a whisper. We're not just flipping a switch: we're reversing the hardware, rewiring the system, and restoring balance.

That's why a nerve block that technically wears off after eight hours can produce changes that last for months or even years. It's not only numbing pain—it's giving your body the chance to undo the damage, to heal from the inside out, to find equilibrium again.

The results? They're nothing short of breathtaking. I've had patients tell me the world suddenly feels alive again. That they're seeing color for the first time in years. That food tastes better, and music moves them.

That they took their first deep breath in over a decade—and sometimes, that one breath is all it takes to begin again.

One veteran told me it was the first time he'd truly been able to take a deep breath since his trauma. The sense of doom—the feeling that something terrible is always just around the corner—evaporates. Instead of living in a state of hypervigilance, they can simply focus. One patient described it like this: "I'm not looking for an attack anymore. I'm just looking. I can actually see what's in front of me."

Some even get their emotions back. I remember a Vietnam vet, a man who hadn't felt a single emotion in thirty years. After the block, he sat in my office and cried like a baby for half an hour. When I asked him what was happening, he looked at me, tears streaming down his face, and said, "I feel something for the first time in decades."

The stellate ganglion block isn't just a treatment: It's a key to unlocking the body's natural ability to heal, to prune away the overgrowth of trauma, and to bring someone back to life—not just surviving, but truly living again.

Because it has a unique quality—it travels along nerve pathways with precision, almost like it's cruising down a neural highway. Scientists took advantage of this by tagging the rabies virus with a fluorescent marker and injecting it into the stellate ganglion of a rat. Then, they waited to see where it would go.

After giving the virus time to travel, the researchers examined the rat's brain—and what they discovered was remarkable. The virus had spread to the amygdala, hippocampus, and hypothalamus—regions of the brain deeply involved in processing fear, emotion, and memory. In other words, the same circuits hijacked in PTSD. This wasn't just theoretical. It was visual, biological proof: the stellate ganglion has a direct line to the very parts of the brain responsible for the trauma response. That means when we target it, we're not just numbing a nerve in the neck—we're sending a powerful signal upstream to the emotional command center of the brain.

So why does this matter for my work? Because this study offers more than theory—it delivers biological proof of a direct line between the stellate ganglion and the brain regions most affected by trauma. When we perform a stellate ganglion block, we're not only calming a local nerve—we're hitting the circuit breaker that controls the most reactive parts of the brain. We're disrupting the signal that keeps someone trapped in survival mode.

The local anesthetic used in the procedure travels through these pathways and immediately begins to quiet the amygdala—one of the brain's key players in the fight-or-flight response. That's why so many patients feel a shift almost instantly: less anxiety, fewer intrusive thoughts, a sense of calm they haven't felt in years.

And as we discussed earlier, trauma triggers the release of nerve growth factor (NGF), a protein that causes sympathetic nerves to sprout extra branches—like an overgrown tree with too many limbs. Each new branch becomes another channel for stress to move through, reinforcing the trauma response. It's like adding more lanes to a highway already flooded with traffic. This same study helped us understand that the stellate ganglion block lowers NGF levels, which in turn causes those extra branches to shrink back. This process—what we call neural pruning—helps restore the system to a calmer, more functional baseline.

We have the data, the imaging, the patient stories, the rabies tracing study, the NGF research, and the long-term outcomes—they all fit together like pieces of a puzzle to reveal one clear truth: the stellate ganglion block doesn't just provide temporary relief, it reaches into the root of PTSD and turns down the volume on a system that's been screaming for far too long. Even Dr. Michael Alkire's research, presented at the American Society of Anesthesiology in 2015, used advanced brain imaging to show that the stellate ganglion block (SGB) can reduce activity in the amygdala.

Now, even with evidence like this—clear biological mechanisms, brain imaging, measurable outcomes—there are still those who ask, "What if it's just a placebo effect?" And honestly? I welcome the question. Because anyone in medicine will tell you: going up against placebo is the ultimate test. If your treatment can't outperform the body's natural ability to heal through belief alone, then you've got work to do.

Well, what if I told you that there are experiments out there that have successfully reversed PTSD in rats and dogs? Sounds wild, right? But it's true.

In this study, researchers wanted to explore whether the stellate ganglion block could really have the kind of profound impact that we'd seen in humans, but in a controlled, scientifically rigorous way. And rats, being the workhorses of experimental science, were the chosen subjects. Buckle up, rat lovers—this one gets a bit gnarly. Just remember, I'm just the messenger here; I read the study, but I didn't actually participate in it.[14]

But before we get into the results, the first question you might ask is, "How do you even give PTSD to a rat?" I mean, it's not like you can sit them down, tell them about world atrocities, and watch them spiral into anxiety. Instead, scientists came up with something just as unpleasant: the good old "rat waterboarding" method. The technical term is the "forced swim test," but let's we can call it what it really is—rat waterboarding.

Essentially, they put the rat into a container of water with no way out. The rat has to keep swimming until it's completely exhausted, and eventually, it gives up, starts to sink, and at the last possible moment, it gets rescued. This repeated stress creates what we call "learned helplessness"—a fancy term for the rat believing that no matter what it does, it's doomed. This is how you replicate the mental state of PTSD in a rat. It's grim, but effective.

Now that we've got our traumatized rat, things get really interesting. Scientists decided to see if they could actually reverse the effects of this induced trauma. So, they divided the rats into two groups: one group received a procedure to block the fight-or-flight nerves—essentially the rat equivalent of the stellate ganglion block (SGB) we use in humans

---

[14] Lohr, J. B., Palmer, B. W., Eidt, C. A., Aailaboyina, S., Mausbach, B. T., Wolkowitz, O. M., Thorp, S. R., & Jeste, D. V. (2015). Is Post-Traumatic Stress Disorder Associated with Premature Senescence? A Review of the Literature. American Journal of Geriatric Psychiatry, 23(7), 709–725. https://doi.org/10.1016/j.jagp.2015.04.001

today. The other group got no treatment at all, just to see the natural progression of trauma without intervention.

The untreated rats, sadly, just gave up. They sank, caught in the same loop of helplessness as before. The rats that had received the nerve block swam like little furry Michael Phelps wannabes, hopped out of the water, and went back to doing whatever it is that happy rats do. They weren't afraid of drowning anymore because that fight-or-flight response had been reset.

What this experiment revealed was nothing short of astonishing: undeniable proof that this isn't just a placebo effect. Let's be real—rats (and dogs like Max) don't do placebos. They aren't pondering their emotional well-being or buying into some experimental hype. They have zero expectations about injections, no hopeful self-talk about turning their lives around. This isn't about belief or mindset; it's pure, unfiltered biology. When you dial down the fight-or-flight response at its core, the changes are real, immediate, and lasting.

But here's where it gets even more fascinating: the study also shows us that PTSD isn't just about memories or psychological conditioning—it's a biological wound, etched into the wiring of the nervous system. And this is exactly what the SGB and DSR does for humans. It's not about coping better or pushing through; it's about going in and resetting the system, like rebooting a computer caught in an endless error loop. Once that fight-or-flight circuit is turned off, the constant fear melts away, hypervigilance quiets down, and you can finally start living again. The treated rats didn't stop acting traumatized because of some good vibes; they changed because those overactive nerve pathways—the ones keeping them stuck in high alert—were switched off. We flipped the biological breaker, and just like that, they found their way back to balance.

There are countless more studies—some completed, many still ongoing—that continue to deepen our understanding of how this works. Research has shown changes in brain activity, shifts in hormone levels, downregulation of inflammatory markers, and clear physiological indicators that this treatment is not only real, but measurable, repeatable, and lasting.

I didn't start out trying to rewrite the book on trauma. I was just trying to help people who had run out of options—people who had been told to manage, cope, and accept a life of constant reactivity. But the more I studied, the more I listened, the more I treated, one thing became undeniable: this works. But these breakthroughs were only the beginning.

What I didn't know then was just how much resistance we'd face trying to bring this treatment into the mainstream. The idea that PTSD could be treated as a physical injury—that you could inject a local anesthetic into a nerve bundle and fundamentally shift how someone processes trauma—shattered the conventional model. It threatened long-standing beliefs. And let's be honest: the medical community doesn't like being challenged. Especially not by something that works outside their expected lines. There were questions, doubts, and pushback, even from those who should've been allies. Even from those who claimed to want the same outcome: healing.

In the chapters ahead, I'll take you inside that battle—how we fought to redefine trauma not as a disorder of weakness, but as a treatable injury of the nervous system. I believe it's important for people to see behind the scenes of what it really takes to drive change. What it means to hold the truth in your hands...while being told, again and again, that it can't possibly be real.

And why we kept going anyway.

CHAPTER 10

ONE LETTER CAN SAVE LIVES

As I continued my work and witnessed the profound impact of the SGB procedure on people grappling with trauma, I found myself stepping into a role beyond that of a doctor: I became a teacher.

Every patient who sat in my office had a story, and often, that story carried an undercurrent of confusion, shame, or hopelessness. They'd been told—or had come to believe—that their struggles were purely psychological, that their trauma was an intangible, elusive ghost haunting their minds. My job wasn't just to treat them; it was to help them understand what was really happening inside their bodies. I would often begin with a simple truth: trauma isn't just in your mind—it lives in your body, including your brain. I'd talk about the physiological changes triggered by trauma, how the nervous system becomes locked in a state of hypervigilance, and how this state can drive the symptoms they were experiencing. I used metaphors to make it relatable, likening their trauma to a car engine stuck in overdrive or a smoke alarm that wouldn't stop blaring, even though the fire had long been extinguished. It was fascinating to watch the lightbulb moments, those instances when the weight of self-blame and confusion lifted, replaced by understanding. For the first time, they saw their trauma not as a mysterious emotional flaw but as a physical condition—one that could be treated, even healed.

As I began treating more Special Forces operators and military veterans, I noticed a recurring theme: Many of them would refer to their struggles as "PTSD," wearing the diagnosis like an invisible badge of dishonor. They felt burdened by the idea that they were somehow broken, living with a "disorder" that might define them for life. Once again, I found myself putting on that teacher hat, explaining that what they were experiencing wasn't a disorder in the traditional sense. Their trauma wasn't a permanent lifestyle or identity—it was a physiological wound. And like any wound, it could be treated and healed. Time and again, I'd see the weight on their shoulders begin to ease as they realized their condition wasn't an untouchable curse, but something tangible and fixable.

It was during this time that I was introduced to a man named Dr. Frank Ochberg. Frank is nothing short of remarkable—a pioneer in understanding trauma and its profound effects. In the 1970s, he was the first to define the term Stockholm syndrome, a designation that reshaped how law enforcement and psychologists approached hostage situations. He crafted it for the FBI and Scotland Yard negotiators, laying the groundwork for modern psychotraumatology.[15] Then, in 1980, Frank took on another monumental task: he was part of the committee that officially named and defined "post-traumatic stress disorder" (PTSD) for the *Diagnostic and Statistical Manual of Mental Disorders (DSM).*

At the time, the term "disorder" seemed like the right fit, offering a language to describe the wounds carried by veterans and trauma survivors. But as the years passed and technology revealed more about how trauma changes the brain and body, Frank's perspective began to shift. Advances in neuroscience and a deeper understanding of the nervous system painted a more complex picture—one that challenged the idea of trauma as a psychological disorder. Instead, Frank began to see it for what it truly was: a physiological injury. By the 1990s, he coined the term "post-traumatic stress injury," (PTSI), and began advocating for this critical paradigm shift.

---

15 Frank M. Ochberg, "The Ties That Bind Captive to Captor," *Los Angeles Times*, April 8, 2005, https://www.latimes.com/archives/la-xpm-2005-apr-08-oe-ochberg8-story.html.

Frank's work wasn't just academic or theoretical—it was revolutionary. He understood that words have power, and how we label something can shape how we perceive, treat, and recover from it. The term "injury" carried with it an inherent promise of healing, a possibility of recovery, and a rejection of the stigma that comes with the word "disorder."

Meeting Frank was like having a door swung wide open to a world of clarity, and his insights gave me the language to describe what I had been intuitively treating in my patients all along. Trauma, as Frank so eloquently argued, wasn't a defect in the individual—it was an injury to their system, one that could be treated, healed, and overcome.

After meeting Frank, it was as though someone had finally handed me the missing piece of a puzzle I'd been wrestling with for years. I had always been uneasy with the term *disorder*; it felt heavy, wrong, like a label slapped onto people to mark them as irreparably broken. When a patient sits across from you, carrying the weight of a diagnosis like PTSD, you can see it in their eyes—the belief that this label defines them, that it's permanent, and that there's no way out. They internalize it, as though it's etched into their identity. And for years, my role as a doctor—and as a teacher—was to dismantle that belief. To show them that what they were dealing with wasn't some nebulous defect in their character, but a physiological response to an overwhelming event. When Frank said the word *injury*, everything snapped into place. This wasn't a new revelation; it was a validation of what I had been explaining to my patients, day after day, year after year.

Unlike *disorder*, which carries the connotation of permanence, *injury* implies something external—something that happened to you, not something that defines you. It shifts the narrative entirely. When someone hears "injury," they don't feel shame—they feel hope. It's a term that invites action: treatment, repair, recovery. Suddenly, trauma isn't a life sentence—it's a challenge your body is built to overcome. Think about it: when you break a bone, you don't internalize it as a personal failure. You don't wonder if you're inherently flawed or if you'll carry that brokenness forever. You seek treatment. You reset the bone, put it in a cast, and trust that it will heal with time and care. That's what the word *injury* offers to those grappling with trauma—a pathway out. It removes the stigma, replacing it with validation and the expectation of recovery.

Dr. Frank Ochberg, a man whose career had already reshaped the understanding of trauma on a global scale, didn't stop at defining terms like Stockholm syndrome or helping to introduce PTSD into the *DSM* back in the '80s. His work didn't just sit in textbooks or FBI training manuals—it continued to evolve with the times, as did his understanding of trauma. And through a series of connections that only someone as deeply entrenched in the field as Frank could have, he found himself allied with a powerhouse in the military world: US Army retired four-star general Peter Chiarelli. General Chiarelli was no stranger to high stakes. Over the course of his nearly forty-year career, he had led the day-to-day operations of the US Army, overseeing 1.1 million soldiers, and had commanded over 147,000 US and Coalition troops in Iraq. But it was during his tenure as vice chief of staff of the Army, from 2008 to 2012, that Chiarelli found himself tasked with what he would later call one of his most challenging missions: addressing the skyrocketing rates of post-traumatic stress (PTS), traumatic brain injuries (TBI), and suicides among soldiers.

Chiarelli's approach was clear-eyed and deeply empathetic. He spent hours in the field, talking to soldiers face-to-face, listening to their struggles, and hearing what they weren't saying. One thing became glaringly obvious: the stigma surrounding PTSD was keeping people from seeking help. The term "disorder" wasn't just a word—it was a weapon. It made soldiers feel weak, like they'd failed before they'd even begun to fight for their recovery. "Disorder" implied something preexisting, something broken inside them, and it created a wall between them and the care they so desperately needed. Chiarelli knew words mattered. In an interview with *PBS NewsHour* in 2011, he said that the term "disorder" perpetuated a bias against the condition, and it made the person seem weak. For a soldier, the ultimate insult is to be labeled weak. The solution, in Chiarelli's mind, was simple but profound: drop the "D." Call it an injury, because an injury, after all, is something that happens to you—not something inherently wrong with you.[16] This perspective wasn't just a military mindset—it was a scientific one, backed by decades of research, and one that resonated deeply with Dr. Frank Ochberg. Together, they began to push for a formal name change: PTSD would become PTSI, post-traumatic stress injury. It was more than a semantic shift; it was a paradigm shift. It had the potential to change everything, from how people viewed themselves to how they sought care. When I learned about their mission, I didn't hesitate—I joined forces with them.

Most people aren't familiar with how medical terminology has evolved over time or why it matters so much—but it's incredibly important that you are. It's a history that can be both fascinating and, at times, downright odd. Medicine's evolution is littered with bizarre, sometimes dark chapters that reflect just how much our understanding—and our language—has shaped the way we view the human condition.

First, let's look at a few comical examples. Take "honey urine," for example. It's not the name of some quaint delicacy, but the term once used to describe diabetes mellitus. In an age without modern diagnostics, physicians would literally taste a patient's urine to confirm its sweetness. Yes, you heard that right—they *tasted* it. As absurd as it sounds now, it's a vivid reminder of how rudimentary knowledge shaped language, and how language, in turn, shaped perception. Tuberculous lymphadenitis was once referred to as "the king's evil" in Europe. The condition, characterized by swollen lymph nodes in the neck, was believed to be curable by the royal touch. Monarchs across Europe would ceremoniously lay hands on those afflicted, wielding supposed divine healing powers until the eighteenth century.

Then there's what we now know as phlegmasia alba dolens in the femoral vein, often occurring postpartum. It caused inflammation that left limbs pale, swollen, and excruciatingly painful—a condition known as "milk leg" or "white leg." Why milk? Probably because someone thought a pale, lifeless limb bore an uncanny resemblance to dairy. And

16 "Army General Calls for Changing Name for PTSD," *PBS NewsHour*, archived November 5, 2011, at https://web.archive.org/web/20111105190417/http://www.pbs.org/newshour/updates/military/july-dec11/stress_11-04.html.

let's not forget "housemaid's knee," the old name for prepatellar bursitis—a condition caused by prolonged kneeling that inflamed the area in front of the kneecap. It may sound quaint, but the name reflects a time when housemaids bore the brunt of hard labor, often without the luxury of modern ergonomic aids.

Eventually, medicine traded in these colorful and sometimes mystical names for a more standardized approach. In 1952, the American Psychiatric Association introduced the first edition of the *Diagnostic and Statistical Manual of Mental Disorders (DSM).* It was a groundbreaking moment, moving psychiatry from informal descriptors to a consistent, clinical framework. This wasn't just a book—it was a system for accurately diagnosing mental health conditions, complete with a glossary of terms. The *DSM* represented a monumental step forward, replacing the age of royal cures and poetic misnomers with a foundation rooted in science and clinical rigor.

But not all of its classifications were triumphs of enlightenment—some were profound failures, leaving scars that resonate even today. Take, for instance, the classification of homosexuality as a mental disorder—a glaring injustice and a black mark on the history of modern psychiatry. For decades, the *DSM* labeled homosexuality as a *mental* defect, an affliction to be "cured." It wasn't just an error; it was a weaponized misunderstanding, one that legitimized cruelty and fueled systemic oppression. This wasn't medicine—it was a moral failure disguised as science, reinforcing stigma and enabling so-called "treatments" that inflicted immeasurable harm on countless lives. The methods were horrific—electric shocks, nausea-inducing drugs, and forced "dates" with young nurses—all in a twisted attempt to force men into heterosexuality. It was the kind of dehumanization that didn't just fail to "cure" anyone; it scarred people, reinforcing shame and stigma. And remember, this wasn't some fringe practice: It was endorsed by the medical establishment until 1973, when the American Psychiatric Association (APA) voted to remove homosexuality from the *DSM*. Even then, the victory was incomplete, because the APA replaced it with a new term: "sexual orientation disturbance," as if the problem lay in the individual's struggle to accept their identity. It wasn't until 1987 (nearly two decades later) that homosexuality was fully erased from the *DSM*'s pages.

Throughout much of history, medical diagnoses have been wielded not as tools for healing, but as weapons of control—especially against women. Take *nymphomania*, for example: what today would be recognized as a healthy sexual desire was once pathologized as a mental illness. In the nineteenth century, women who expressed even moderate sexual agency could be slapped with the label of *nymphomaniac* and deemed unfit for society. Husbands and fathers wielded this diagnosis like a gavel, committing their wives and daughters to asylums for behaviors that, in men, would have been celebrated. It wasn't about medicine; it was about control. Once institutionalized, these women faced horrifying treatments: isolation, forced celibacy, and even surgical interventions like the removal of ovaries or clitorises were common, all justified under the pseudoscience of the day. The underlying message was clear: female sexuality, if it didn't conform to societal norms, was something to be feared, controlled, and eradicated.

And then there was *hysteria*—the ultimate catch-all diagnosis for any woman who dared to step outside the narrow boundaries of acceptable femininity. Derived from the Greek word *hystera*, meaning "uterus," this "diagnosis" was built on the absurd belief that a woman's reproductive organs were the root of her emotional instability. Fainting? Hysteria. Irritability? Hysteria. Expressing anger, sadness, sexual desire, or—God forbid—disagreeing with her husband? Definitely hysteria. Women labeled "hysterical" weren't just dismissed—they were institutionalized, silenced, and stripped of their autonomy. Their crime? Speaking out. Seeking independence. Refusing to conform. And men held all the power. A husband or father could have a woman committed for practically any reason—too outspoken, too emotional, too inconvenient. Once inside the system, the implications were devastating.

Some were sentenced to what was called the "rest cure"—a kind of medical house arrest that confined women to bed and forbade reading, writing, or even conversation. The goal was enforced passivity, total dependence, and psychological submission. For those deemed more severe, the treatment escalated: electroshock therapy, and in some cases, lobotomies. A little farther back in history, physicians believed the uterus could literally *wander* around the body, causing chaos wherever it went. The solution? Scent therapy—also known as fumigation. They'd place pleasant fragrances near a woman's genitals to lure the uterus back to its "proper" place, while holding foul odors under her nose to drive it downward. Sneezing was sometimes induced as a kind of internal reset. It was invasive, it was degrading, and it was all based on pseudoscience dressed up as medicine.

The women subjected to this weren't just failed by the system—they were erased by it. Women who might have been leaders, artists, healers, or visionaries were reduced to patients, pathologized for being too alive in a world that demanded they be quiet. These diagnoses didn't just hurt individual women—they upheld an entire societal structure that equated obedience with health, and defiance with disease. It's important to understand this—not just for the history lesson, but because medical paradigms evolve. They always have. And sometimes the most dangerous ones aren't the most dramatic. They're the ones so embedded in the system that no one thinks to question them. Until someone does.

The legacies of *nymphomania* and *hysteria* still haunt us. While both diagnoses have been retired (hysteria was finally removed from the *DSM* in 1980), their echoes remain in how women's autonomy and emotions are sometimes dismissed today. These terms weren't just bad science: they were tools of the patriarchy, used to enforce submission and strip women of agency. What makes this history so chilling is how easily it happened. Medicine, the very field meant to heal and protect, became a vehicle for societal control. It's a stark reminder that labels matter. The way we name and understand mental and physical conditions can shape not just treatment but the way people see themselves—and how society sees them.

Think about it: the absurdity of "honey urine" feels almost quaint now, a harmless relic of medicine's more colorful past. But the legacy of calling homosexuality a disorder or labeling women as hysterical is far from benign—it's a reminder of how devastating language can be when it stigmatizes and dehumanizes. These aren't just outdated words; they're markers of a time when medicine failed to see the whole person. They represent a failure to understand, a failure to care, and, worst of all, a denial of dignity. They stand as cautionary tales of how deeply flawed terminology can harm—not only by misdiagnosing but by perpetuating suffering.

As I joined forces with Dr. Frank Ochberg and US General Peter Chiarelli, I realized we were embarking on another such moment in history. This was our chance to make things right—to rewrite the narrative around trauma in a way that restored dignity and opened the door to healing. With Frank's groundbreaking contributions to defining trauma and Pete's tireless advocacy for reducing stigma within the military, we knew the stakes were high.

I started with a deep dive into the history of the term "PTSD," peeling back the layers to understand how it came to be. The history of trauma is as old as humanity itself, etched into our myths, wars, and the ways we've tried—and often failed—to heal invisible wounds. Long before medical manuals and clinical diagnoses, stories like Homer's *Iliad* captured the haunting effects of battle. Achilles, the mighty warrior, wasn't just a hero: he was a man tormented by grief and rage after the death of his closest companion. His withdrawal from the battlefield wasn't just strategy—it was trauma, the kind we now recognize but struggled for centuries to name.

As societies evolved, so too did the labels we gave to the scars left by catastrophic events. In the 1600s, soldiers who longed for home were said to suffer from "nostalgia," a term that painted their despair as homesickness rather than something more profound. During the American Civil War, doctors observed veterans plagued by rapid heartbeats, anxiety, and debilitating fatigue. They called it "soldier's heart," believing the condition stemmed from cardiac issues. These terms acknowledged suffering but fell short of understanding its cause.

With the rise of industrialization came new kinds of trauma. Survivors of catastrophic train accidents were said to have "railway spine," a condition doctors attributed to physical damage from the violent jarring of the body. The idea that emotional distress could manifest physically wasn't yet understood, so the mind and body were treated as separate. The language reflected this disconnect, leaving sufferers misunderstood and often dismissed.

The horrors of World War I changed everything. Soldiers exposed to relentless shelling began exhibiting tremors, emotional numbness, and an inability to speak or function. The term "shell shock" emerged, rooted in the belief that exposure to exploding shells caused physical damage to the brain. But as more cases appeared among soldiers without physical injuries, it became evident that the root cause was physiological. Even so, the stigma was brutal. Men were labeled cowards, shamed for their perceived weakness, or sent back into battle with little understanding of the toll war had taken on their minds.

World War II brought more refined terms like "combat fatigue" and "battle fatigue," reflecting an acknowledgment of the strain prolonged warfare placed on soldiers. But while these names edged closer to recognizing trauma's psychological impact, they didn't erase the stigma. Veterans returned home carrying the weight of their experiences, often left to cope in silence.

After the Vietnam War, soldiers came back not only scarred by combat but also alienated by a divided nation that offered neither welcome nor understanding. They endured flashbacks, nightmares, emotional numbness, and hypervigilance, but their symptoms were dismissed under the label "Vietnam syndrome."

By 1980, the medical community finally took a significant step forward. Post-traumatic stress disorder was formally recognized in the third edition of the *DSM*: *DSM-III*. For the first time, trauma was categorized as a legitimate mental health condition, not a moral failing or a weakness of character. This change wasn't just academic—it was a lifeline, offering veterans and survivors of other traumas a framework to understand what they were experiencing and a path toward treatment.

Cultures across the globe have always had their ways of describing the invisible scars left by war. Russian soldiers returning from the brutal conflict in Chechnya were said to suffer from "Chechnya syndrome," just as Americans labeled the struggles of Vietnam veterans as "Vietnam syndrome." It's clear to us now that this wasn't about the geography. Trauma doesn't carry a flag. It wasn't some isolated curse striking soldiers in one corner of the world or another. No, there is a clear pattern emerging, like a neon sign flashing in the darkness: this is bigger than any one war, any one group of people. For decades, we fumbled to name it, as though each conflict had birthed its own mysterious affliction. But the truth can't be boxed into neat little categories. This isn't about the location; it's about the shared human experience of living through hell and trying to come out the other side.

The journey from Homer's Achilles to the formal recognition of PTSD is a story of humanity grappling with the unseen scars of life. It's a reminder that trauma isn't new—it's as old as war, loss, and disaster itself. And while the names we've given it have often failed to capture its depth, each step forward has brought us closer to understanding and healing the wounds we cannot see with naked eye. This is why the push to reframe PTSD as PTSI matters so profoundly. Language shapes how we perceive the world and ourselves. With one word, we have the chance to dismantle stigma, offer hope, and transform the way trauma survivors see their condition. History has taught us the dangers of getting this wrong—of clinging to harmful labels that trap people in shame. But it has also shown us the extraordinary power of getting it right.

Dr. Frank Ochberg and General Peter Chiarelli understood this, and so did I. Trauma isn't some inherent flaw or defect in a person—it's a physiological and emotional response to an external event. By redefining it as an injury, we're not just slapping a new label on the same thing; we're reframing the entire story around trauma. We're telling people: *This is real. This is treatable. And you're not broken beyond repair.* That shift, as small as it might seem to an outsider, has the power to change lives. For someone who feels defined by their trauma, hearing that it's an injury—not a disorder—can feel like someone handing them a lifeline.

So, we rolled up our sleeves, ready to fight for this change. To change a diagnostic name, you have to prove the existing one causes harm—like stigma. That's why "learning disabilities" became "learning differences."

With great passion and determination, I threw my support behind the movement to make PTSI the new standard. Alongside Frank, General Chiarelli, and a growing coalition of voices, we aimed to challenge the entrenched stigma that had caused so much unnecessary suffering. We made our case with everything we had. I submitted my institutional review board survey with the facts laid out in stark, undeniable terms: the weight of a single word, the stigma it carried, the lives lost to suicide because of what that label implied. This wasn't just about semantics—it was about the very real, measurable harm perpetuated by a diagnosis that told people they were broken, disordered, and beyond repair.

It was all on the table, plain as day. And the response from the American Psychiatric Association APA, the gatekeepers of the *DSM*? A bureaucratic shrug and three dismissive words: "Not enough information." That was it. Case closed. Their message couldn't have been clearer: *To change the name, you must prove beyond all doubt that the current name is harmful.* And in their eyes, we hadn't done enough. The subtext? *Come back when you have more data—or don't bother coming back at all.*

I was stunned. We'd built an airtight argument, presented a clear-cut case, and demonstrated the life-and-death stakes of this decision. But they weren't budging. And as I sat there, dumbfounded, I realized something critical: they weren't just clinging to outdated terminology because of tradition or oversight. There was more at play—something far more insidious. The truth is there's a lot of money tied to the word "disorder."

A disorder implies something chronic, something you'll live with forever. And that narrative? It's a pharmaceutical goldmine. If someone believes they're inherently broken, that their condition is a lifelong sentence, they're much easier to sell on a lifetime of medication. Pills for the symptoms. Pills for the side effects of the first pills. Pills to help you cope with the idea that you'll always need pills.

But the term *injury?* That's different. An injury suggests something treatable, something temporary. It suggests the possibility of real recovery—of putting down the pills, stepping out of the system, and walking away whole. And for an industry built on perpetual treatment rather than cure, that's not a narrative they're eager to embrace. The push to rename PTSD to PTSI wasn't just an idea—it was backed by science and the lived experiences of countless individuals.

I wasn't going to give up easily. If we were going to challenge the system, we needed more than passion—we needed proof. So, I led a study to measure what a name change could actually mean. This wasn't about tossing around ideas in a vacuum. It was about listening to the people who mattered most—the ones living with trauma—and giving the APA the "data," they kept demanding. We launched an anonymous global survey through the Stella Center, an organization dedicated to treating emotional trauma and redefining mental health care. The goal was simple: find out how language was shaping reality.

Between August 2021 and August 2022, the survey was distributed to 3,000 participants: 1,500 were clinic patients and visitors, while the other 1,500 were website visitors. The goal was to gauge whether changing the name from PTSD to PTSI could reduce stigma, improve hope, and increase the likelihood of seeking treatment. Over 1,000 people completed the survey, and the findings were striking. More than two-thirds of respondents believed that the term "PTSI" would reduce stigma. Over half said it would give them more hope for finding a solution and make them more likely to seek medical help. The impact was particularly profound among those who had been diagnosed with PTSD—they were the ones most likely to believe in the transformative potential of the name change.

The data also revealed how stigma acts as a barrier to care. Nearly 41.2 percent of adults with PTSD experience self-stigmatization—internalizing negative stereotypes about their condition, which prevents them from seeking the help they desperately need. And this isn't just about mental distress: Untreated PTSD is linked to increased rates of suicide, domestic violence, and other devastating outcomes. It's a condition that ripples outward, affecting families, communities, and entire societies. The study showed that changing the name to PTSI could help dismantle these barriers. Participants expressed that the new term would not only improve their likelihood of seeking medical help but also make them more open to innovative treatments like the SGB or transcranial magnetic stimulation (TMS). The data was clear: this shift could change lives.

Despite presenting compelling evidence, the push to change the name from PTSD to PTSI hit a wall of resistance. The APA dismissed the proposal with a clinical shrug, citing a lack of sufficient evidence even after presenting conclusive evidence. It was disheartening, to say the least. We had gathered peer-reviewed studies, expert testimonies, and survey data directly from the people most impacted by trauma—people who had lived with the burden of this label and understood firsthand the power of language to harm or heal. Yet, it wasn't enough.

Their rejection felt like more than a bureaucratic decision—it felt like a refusal to listen to the voices of those who desperately needed change. It was a stark reminder of how entrenched systems can be, how difficult it is to shift the tides of an institution that clings to tradition, even when that tradition perpetuates harm. For a moment, it was easy to feel defeated. After all, the evidence was clear: the term "disorder" carried stigma, fed shame, and created barriers to care. Yet, the people in charge of changing it seemed unwilling to budge.

But here's the thing about this fight—it's not just a professional mission, it's deeply personal. It's driven by every single person I've sat across from whose life has been touched by trauma. It's fueled by the voices of warriors, survivors, spouses, first responders, and clinicians who've told me—sometimes in broken sentences, sometimes through tears—that the label "disorder" made them feel defective. Beyond repair. Like there was something wrong with who they were, not something that had happened to them. They've shared how reframing trauma as an injury—something external, treatable, and temporary—restored their sense of dignity, of hope. That simple shift in language created a bridge back to possibility. A belief that they weren't broken—they were wounded. And wounds, with the right care, can heal.

Those voices are what keep us in this fight. They're louder than the resistance. They remind us that we're not pushing for change out of theory or politics—we're pushing because the stakes are human lives. Yes, the red tape is maddening. Yes, the inertia is real. But giving up is not an option. Not when hope is on the line. We know the power of language to shape reality. We've seen how the label "disorder" discourages people from seeking help, how it isolates them, and how it feeds the cycle of stigma that keeps so many trapped in silence. And we've seen how the word "injury" can transform that narrative, opening the door to care, validation, and recovery. The APA may have dismissed our proposal, but that doesn't mean the fight is over. If anything, it's a call to push harder, to gather more evidence, to rally more voices. Change rarely comes easily, especially when it challenges deeply entrenched systems. But history has shown us that persistence pays off. The same resistance was faced when homosexuality was removed from the *DSM*, when terms like hysteria were finally retired, and when countless other outdated classifications were challenged and redefined. Each time, it took people willing to stand up, to push back, and to say, "This isn't right."

That's exactly what we're going to do. The voices of those survey participants—the soldiers, the survivors, the people who have lived with trauma—will not be ignored. Their stories matter. Their experiences matter. And their hope matters. So, we're rolling up our sleeves, gathering more data, building more coalitions, and making it impossible for the APA—or anyone else—to deny the truth. This fight isn't just about changing a word; it's about changing lives. It's about giving people the tools they need to heal, the validation they deserve, and the hope they've been searching for. And no amount of resistance is going to stop us from seeing this mission through. Because when you're fighting for something this important, you don't back down. You dig in, you keep going, and eventually, you win.

I've committed myself to leading this charge for change. I hope, with every fiber of my being, that I'll see it happen in my lifetime. If you visit my website today (dreugenelipov.com), you'll find the ongoing work, the relentless effort to push this forward. The fight isn't over, not by a long shot. I'll continue to wear the hat of teacher alongside doctor, educating one person at a time, even if that's what it takes to make a difference. Because sometimes, one word can change everything. One word can dismantle stigma, open the door to treatment, and give someone the courage to believe in their own healing. One word can save a life. And I won't stop until that word—*injury*—becomes the cornerstone of a future where trauma is no longer a life sentence but a wound that can heal.

CHAPTER 11

LET'S TALK ABOUT PSYCHEDELIC AND ALTERNATIVE THERAPIES

So far, we've been laser focused on a major breakthrough in how we treat trauma—one that challenges everything we've been conditioned to believe about PTSD, the nervous system, and recovery itself. But with any major shift in understanding, big questions inevitably follow. Is this the ultimate cure? Does this mean we don't need any other therapy? Should the SGB replace everything else? And what about alternative therapies? What about psychedelics? Do they work?

These are important questions. Because while the SGB is a powerful tool, one that has changed countless lives, it's not the *only* tool. We are living in an era where more options exist for treating trauma than ever before. That's both exciting…and overwhelming. For every promising breakthrough, there's a flood of opinions, studies, personal testimonies, and contradictions.

The truth is, we're drowning in information. One person swears by a treatment, calling it life-changing; another claims that same treatment will fry your brain and ruin your life. And in the age of social media, we don't just have experts—we have *self-appointed* experts. People with no real background in medicine, neuroscience, or trauma therapy, who have taken it upon themselves to educate the masses. And the internet eats it up. The louder and more dramatic the claim, the more attention it gets. The truth is, not all treatments are created equal. Some are groundbreaking, some are useless, and some teeter between being revolutionary and reckless.

The truth is, SGB isn't the only answer—and it was never meant to be. As powerful as it is, I've seen it work best when it's not treated as a standalone cure, but as a *catalyst*—something that unlocks the system so other healing modalities can actually take root. That's where this chapter comes in: It's time to talk about alternative therapies. And no, I don't mean throwing a dozen trendy tools at the wall and hoping one sticks. The goal here isn't to chase novelty—it's to ask better questions. To look critically at what actually works. To understand *why* so many people are looking beyond conventional treatment in the first place.

Because that's the real question, isn't it? Why do we need alternative therapies at all? By definition, alternative therapies exist outside the mainstream—they're what people turn to when the "approved" routes leave them stuck. When the gold standard doesn't deliver gold results. When the standard of care feels more like standard *coping* than true healing. So, before we explore what's out there, we need to take a step back and look at what these "alternatives" are actually an alternative *to.*

What does conventional PTSD treatment really look like? What's the dominant model that psychiatry and medicine keep pushing forward? And perhaps the most important question of all: *If the current system works, why are so many people still suffering?* We've poured billions into mental health. Entire industries have been built around managing a lifestyle of trauma. And yet…here we are. With rising suicide rates, people stuck on medications that numb but never heal, and survivors shuffled from one therapist to the next, reliving their trauma but never feeling whole again.

This chapter isn't about bashing the system—it's about *naming its limits.* Because when we understand the limitations of conventional treatment—what it gets right, what it gets terribly wrong—we can finally see why so many are seeking something different. Not out of desperation, but out of discernment. So, let's start there—with a hard look at the current model: its pillars, its promises, and the quiet failures that brought us to the edge of something new. Only then can we talk about what comes next.

In traditional medicine, PTSD treatment relies on two primary pillars: psychotherapy and pharmaceuticals. These form the gold standard of care—the officially endorsed, government-approved, and insurance-backed methods required by institutions like the VA. Walk into a VA clinic with PTSD, and chances are, these will be your only options. Let's break that down, starting with psychotherapy.

Psychotherapy

Psychotherapy is a broad term, and within it, several approaches exist, some more effective than others. These fall into two main categories:

Cognitive Behavioral Therapy (CBT)

CBT is the therapy world's Swiss Army knife—widely used for everything from anxiety to depression to PTSD. The idea is simple: your thoughts shape your reality, so if you can change your thoughts, you can change your life. Sounds good, right? In theory, sure. CBT for PTSD focuses on identifying and restructuring negative thought patterns that keep people stuck in a loop of fear, avoidance, and emotional distress. The goal is to help someone recognize distorted beliefs about their trauma—*"I am broken," "I'll never be safe," "It was my fault"*—and replace them with more rational, constructive ones.

Does it work? For some people, absolutely. But let's be real: telling someone who has just survived a warzone, a mass shooting, or years of abuse that they need to *reframe their thinking* can feel a bit like handing a drowning man a book on swimming techniques. It's helpful in the long run, but as an intervention? Not for everyone.

Cognitive Processing Therapy (CPT)

A close cousin of CBT, CPT takes things a step further, focusing specifically on reprocessing the traumatic event itself. This means breaking down how the trauma changed the person's beliefs about themselves, the world, and others—and then challenging those beliefs.

Think of it as a mental excavation process: *Why do you believe you're unsafe? Why do you think you were responsible for what happened? How has this trauma reshaped the way you see the world?* By systematically unpacking these thoughts, CPT aims to help people move past the rigid, trauma-driven beliefs that keep them locked in a state of hypervigilance and emotional pain.

Again, great in theory. But in practice? It can feel like an intellectual exercise rather than something that actually heals the *physiological* wounds of trauma. And when someone's nervous system is stuck in fight-or-flight mode, just talking about their trauma over and over doesn't reset the body's stress response. Because here's the unfortunate truth: *forcing someone to relive their trauma without properly addressing the physiological damage that trauma has caused?* That can actually make things worse. Think of it like throwing someone into an ice-cold lake to teach them how to swim: some will figure it out; others will drown. And when it comes to PTSD, drowning looks like worsening symptoms, emotional shutdown, or straight-up abandoning therapy altogether.

To be clear, psychotherapy isn't useless. For some people, it's exactly what they need. It can be a powerful space for insight and connection. But let's not pretend it works for everyone.

First, it relies on verbal processing—which doesn't always align with how trauma actually lives in the body. Trauma isn't just a story to be told. It's a physical imprint, a survival loop etched into the nervous system. Talking *about* it doesn't necessarily touch *where* it lives.

Second, it assumes people have the emotional bandwidth to dive into painful memories when, in reality, many are just trying to make it through the day. They're not ready to unpack the past because their system is still locked in survival mode. And finally—and perhaps most critically—it often ignores the body's physiological state entirely. It fails to address how trauma rewires the brain and body at a foundational level. The nervous system has no place in the conversation, and that's a massive oversight.

Because here's the truth: timing matters. For many people, psychotherapy becomes more effective *after* a physiological reset. Once the gas pedal has been released and the body is no longer locked in fight-or-flight, the brain becomes more receptive, the system more stable, and the emotional work more productive. It's not about replacing therapy—it's about sequencing it. If you're dealing with serious trauma, the reset may need to come first. Then the talking can do what it's meant to do. That's the piece so many people miss.

And just as a side note—many of the therapies mentioned above become significantly more effective *after* SGB.

Exposure Therapy

Exposure therapy is built on the idea that avoidance strengthens fear, and repeated exposure to trauma in a controlled setting can help the nervous system relearn that the danger has passed. In theory, it makes sense—like treating a phobia by slowly facing it until the fear fades. The goal is habituation—gradual desensitization to the trauma, so the fight-or-flight response diminishes over time. Some argue it works. I've debated its efficacy with psychiatrists and researchers, including Dr. Edna Foa, a pioneer in prolonged exposure therapy for PTSD. The logic isn't flawed—under the right conditions, with the right therapist, it can help reduce avoidance, lessen distress, and shift the nervous system out of hyperarousal.

But here's the problem: PTSD isn't just an exaggerated fear response—it's a deeply wired physiological reaction. The nervous system has been rewired to expect danger, to stay hypervigilant. Forcing someone to relive their worst moments over and over doesn't necessarily help them process the trauma. For many, it just reinforces it—reactivating the same stress response that keeps them stuck.

I've spoken to countless veterans who said it didn't help—in fact, it made them worse. One told me, *"They basically made me watch the battlefield play on a loop in my head. I already relived it every night—I didn't need their help."* Another said flat-out, *"I don't know a single person who finished it."*

The data backs this up: Dropout rates for prolonged exposure therapy are staggeringly high, and many patients report worsening symptoms. If nearly half the people who try it quit because they can't tolerate it, can we really call it effective? And for some, repeated exposure doesn't heal—it retraumatizes. Instead of teaching the brain, *This isn't happening anymore,* it reinforces, *This is happening all the time.*

So, is exposure therapy the worst option? Maybe not. But it's a high-risk, high-reward gamble that assumes people can withstand an intense process before they've even been given the tools to regulate their nervous system. Success rate is under 20 percent, and when nearly half of them walk away worse than when they started, we have to ask: Is this really the best we can do?

Pharmaceuticals

Alongside psychotherapy, medication is the other dominant approach in conventional PTSD treatment. It's the standard protocol: if you walk into a VA clinic or a psychiatrist's office with PTSD, chances are you'll walk out with a prescription.

The most commonly prescribed medications fall into three primary categories:

> **Selective Serotonin Reuptake Inhibitors (SSRIs)**—Medications like Prozac, Zoloft, and Paxil are commonly used as first-line treatments. They're designed to increase serotonin levels in the brain to help regulate mood.
>
> **Atypical Antipsychotics**—Originally developed for conditions such as schizophrenia or bipolar disorder, drugs like Seroquel and Risperdal are sometimes prescribed

off-label for PTSD to help manage symptoms like anxiety, agitation, or intrusive thoughts.

Benzodiazepines—Medications such as Xanax, Ativan, and Klonopin are fast-acting sedatives prescribed to reduce acute anxiety, panic, or insomnia. They work by enhancing the effect of a neurotransmitter called gamma-aminobutyric acid (GABA), which helps calm brain activity.

These medications are often prescribed individually or in combination, depending on the patient's symptoms and response to treatment. In many clinical settings, pharmaceuticals are used as a core component of a comprehensive PTSD management plan.

And just to be crystal clear: **Please do not stop or change any medications without first consulting your healthcare provider.** The perspectives shared below reflect my personal views and interpretations of existing research. I fully acknowledge that these medications have helped many people, but it's also important to recognize that some carry significant risks. I do not prescribe these medications and do not claim to be an expert in psychopharmacology. What follows is based on previously published studies and is intended to inform and encourage thoughtful exploration, not to replace professional medical advice.

SSRIs

SSRIs are the pharmaceutical world's default setting for PTSD. They work by increasing serotonin levels in the brain, which theoretically helps regulate mood, decrease anxiety, and improve overall emotional stability, in theory. In practice, SSRIs are a Band-Aid at best. They don't heal PTSD—they just blunt some of the symptoms. Here's a few of problems. First, they take weeks to kick in. If you're in crisis, waiting a month to feel maybe a little better isn't exactly helpful. They don't work for everyone. Some people feel a noticeable difference. Others feel nothing. They can have serious side effects—nausea, weight gain, emotional numbness, sexual dysfunction—you name it. And withdrawal is brutal. Stopping SSRIs suddenly can trigger brain zaps, mood swings, dizziness, and even worse anxiety than before.

And the biggest issue? They don't actually treat PTSD—they just take the edge off.

Remember the analogy of the gas pedal? PTSD/PTSI is like having your foot slammed down on the gas pedal with no way to let up. Your nervous system is stuck in overdrive, revving high, running hot. What SSRIs do isn't pull back the gas pedal—they just apply the brake at the same time. So now, instead of being completely out of control, you're in a car that's both speeding up and slamming on the brakes at the same time. You might not be spinning out, but your system is still overloaded, still fighting itself, still stuck in dysfunction. The real problem isn't solved—it's just suppressed.

At best, SSRIs help people function while they do the real work of healing through therapy or other interventions. But at worst? They keep people stuck in survival mode, numbed out just enough to tolerate their pain—but never actually getting better.

Atypical Antipsychotics

If SSRIs are the first line of defense, atypical antipsychotics are the heavy artillery—powerful, sedating, and, in many cases, downright dangerous. Drugs like Risperdal (risperidone) and Seroquel (quetiapine) were originally designed for schizophrenia and severe bipolar disorder; they were never meant to treat PTSD. But somewhere along the way, they became standard practice—especially in the VA system.

Here's the problem: they're essentially *major* tranquilizers. They don't heal PTSD—they just shut everything down. They increase the risk of diabetes. Your blood sugar levels go haywire, and before you know it, you're dealing with a whole new health crisis. They can literally stop your heart. Studies show one in 1,000 users per year experience sudden cardiac arrest. They double or triple suicide risk if you miss doses. That's right—if you forget to take your pill on schedule, your risk of suicide can skyrocket.

Let's pause on that last one for a second. Imagine this: You're struggling with PTSD. You're prescribed an antipsychotic that makes you feel like a zombie. You finally decide to stop taking it—or maybe you just forget a few doses. Suddenly, you're hit with an intense rebound effect: worse anxiety, worse depression, and a significantly increased risk of suicidal thoughts. Let's just say that's not exactly the outcome we're aiming for. And yet, despite all of this, these drugs are handed out like candy to veterans, first responders, and trauma survivors—many of whom have no idea about the risks they're taking.

There are a few side effect that are just scary: diabetes, possible increase in suicide rate, obesity, enlarged male breast tissue, and possible cardiac arrests.

Benzodiazepines

Benzodiazepines—often called "benzos"—are a class of fast-acting sedatives commonly prescribed to manage acute anxiety, panic attacks, and insomnia. They work by enhancing the activity of GABA, a neurotransmitter that slows down brain function and calms the nervous system. This calming effect can provide quick relief in moments of intense distress. Some of the most well-known benzos include Valium (diazepam), Xanax (alprazolam), Ativan (lorazepam), and Klonopin (clonazepam). Because of their rapid onset, they're often used when immediate symptom control is needed.

However, benzos carry serious risks—particularly when used long-term. They are highly habit-forming, and physical dependence can develop in a short amount of time. Stopping suddenly after extended use can trigger withdrawal symptoms ranging from anxiety and insomnia to seizures and, in rare cases, death. Due to these concerns, most medical guidelines recommend benzodiazepines only for short-term use and generally not as a frontline treatment for PTSD. Their use in trauma care remains a point of caution and careful clinical judgment.

So just to recap: traditional PTSD treatment rests on two pillars—psychotherapy and pharmaceuticals. These are the officially endorsed, government-approved, insurance-backed approaches required by institutions like the VA. This is what's considered the "gold standard."

To be clear, medication has its place. Some people genuinely benefit from SSRIs. In certain cases, antipsychotics may be necessary to manage severe agitation or help with sleep. But let's be honest—these aren't cures: They don't reset the nervous system, and they don't reverse the physiological damage that trauma inflicts. What they *do* is sedate, suppress, and stabilize—and sometimes, they do that at a steep cost. And that's the real problem with the conventional PTSD model: it was never designed to heal. It was built to manage. To contain. To keep people just functional enough to get by.

A 2011 study published in *The Journal of the American Medical Association* by Dr. Charles Hoge, a clinical psychiatrist from Walter Reed, revealed just how ineffective this "gold standard" really is in practice.[17] Treatment compliance is shockingly low—not because people don't want to get better, but because the treatments are often too painful, impractical, or ineffective. In clinical trials, dropout rates range from 20 to 40 percent. In real-world settings, they're even higher. And for those who *do* stick with therapy? The actual recovery rate is just 40 percent.

Let's put that into perspective: placebo treatments—doing nothing but thinking you're getting help—have an efficacy rate of 32 percent. That means the best treatments modern psychiatry has to offer are only *marginally* more effective than placebo. Compare that to the outcomes we've seen with SGB, where efficacy rates climb as high as 80 to 85 percent, largely because people actually *stay with it*. The difference isn't just in what works—it's in what people can *actually do*. That matters a lot.

If the most widely recommended approach to PTSD treatment barely works half the time—and even then, still leaves patients dependent on long-term therapy and medication—how exactly can we call this a success? And yet, for decades, this has been the dominant strategy.

---

17 Hoge, Charles W. "Interventions for war-related posttraumatic stress disorder: Meeting veterans where they are." Jama306.5 (2011): 549-551.

No wonder so many people are searching for *alternatives*. That's why it's time to broaden the conversation. We owe it to those struggling with trauma to explore what else is out there. The demand for alternatives isn't coming from nowhere—it's coming from people who have exhausted every conventional option and are still suffering. It's coming from veterans, first responders, survivors of abuse, and countless others who have tried the so-called "gold standard" treatments only to find themselves stuck in the same cycle of pain. This is exactly why we need to have a serious conversation about what's missing from the equation—and what alternative approaches might be able to fill the gaps.

We're about to take a hard look at some of the most talked about alternative therapies—the risks, the rewards, and everything in between. If you're here out of curiosity, you'll probably find the information fascinating. But if you're here because you or someone you love is stuck in the deep end of trauma, you're not interested in philosophical debates. You just want your life back. And that's the real question, isn't it? *How do you know what's right for you?*

That's what the next two chapters are here to help you answer. We're going to lay the groundwork by educating you on what's out there—the most common interventions, how they work, and where they fit. No hype, no fluff—just clarity. Think of it as getting all the blocks on the table. Once you see what's available, you'll be better equipped to make strategic, informed decisions.

Then, in the next chapter, we'll go a step further. I'll walk you through a practical framework to help you construct your own healing path—one that's tailored to your needs, goals, and biology. Because this isn't about chasing every shiny new therapy. It's about finding what works for *you.* I'm not here to give you a diagnosis—I can't do that without knowing you personally. But I *can* give you a clear-eyed, expert perspective to help you cut through the noise and take action. At the end of the day, it's not about gold standards or industry debates. It's about your healing.

Psychedelics

There are a handful of alternative therapies we'll explore, but few are as widely discussed—or as controversial—as psychedelics. These substances have been used for thousands of years across cultures, yet in recent years, they've experienced a dramatic resurgence, particularly in the conversation around PTSD treatment. Once dismissed as counterculture, psychedelics are now being reexamined by research institutions, government agencies, and even the VA—not as recreational drugs, but as potential breakthroughs for trauma recovery.

The same substances that were banned and vilified for decades are now being explored for their ability to reset the nervous system, reprocess trauma, and create lasting psychological change. But with all the excitement comes confusion. Some hail psychedelics as the ultimate breakthrough, a cure for trauma that mainstream medicine has failed to deliver. Others warn of risks, side effects, and lingering unknowns. And in the midst of it all, a flood of self-proclaimed experts and internet warriors have made it harder than ever to separate fact from fiction.

So, what's the truth? How do psychedelics work, and are they actually effective for PTSD? Let's cut through the noise.

A quick look at the history books and we'll see that psychedelics aren't anything new. The Western world may treat them like a groundbreaking discovery, but for thousands of years, civilizations have used these substances for insight, healing, and transformation. Before they were criminalized and dismissed, they were revered as sacred tools—bridges between the seen and unseen, pathways to healing, and ways to understand human consciousness.

A shaman's pouch (dated to more than 1,000 years ago) found in the Andes contained traces of cocaine, psilocin (magic mushrooms), and the base ingredients of ayahuasca—evidence that these substances weren't randomly used: they were carefully selected, understood, and applied. In ancient Mesoamerica, sacred mushrooms were depicted in carvings and ceremonies. The Aztecs called them "teonanácatl"—"fungus of the gods." These weren't just seen as chemicals altering brain function, they were tools for reconnecting with the world and breaking down barriers between individuals, nature, and spirit.

Meanwhile, in ancient Greece, the Eleusinian Mysteries involved kykeon, a psychoactive brew believed to induce profound, life-changing experiences—possibly derived from ergot, a precursor to LSD. Across the world, from Siberian shamans using *Amanita muscaria* to indigenous North Americans consuming peyote, psychedelics were never just about visions—they were woven into the fabric of healing, storytelling, and cultural continuity.

For a brief moment, modern medicine caught on. In the 1950s and early '60s, psychedelics were hailed as breakthrough treatments for alcoholism, depression, and existential distress. Psychotherapists across the US and Europe were using psilocybin and LSD in clinical settings, and early studies were promising—patients reported lasting improvements, reduced anxiety, and even deep, transformative insights.

But then came the cultural revolution of the 1960s. Psychedelics escaped the lab and landed in the hands of the counterculture. LSD became synonymous with rebellion, anti-war protests, and youth movements. Politicians, driven by fear and control rather than science, cracked down. By the mid-1970s, psychedelics were outlawed, research was shut down, and these substances were labeled dangerous and without medical value. Reports of bad trips, psychotic episodes, and hospitalizations only fueled the crackdown, leading to their classification as Schedule I drugs—bringing the era of psychedelic therapy to an abrupt halt. For decades, they remained locked away in the "bad drug" category—despite centuries of historical use and early promising research.

Meanwhile, pharmaceutical companies flooded the market with SSRIs, benzodiazepines, and antipsychotics, offering numbing over healing, suppression over transformation.

Now, the tide is turning. In the past two decades, research institutions like Johns Hopkins, Imperial College London, and the Multidisciplinary Association for Psychedelic Studies have led the charge in studying psilocybin, MDMA, ketamine, and LSD for PTSD, depression, addiction, and existential distress. But this isn't just a repeat of the 1950s—it's a merging of ancient wisdom with modern science.

This resurgence isn't just about how psychedelics affect serotonin receptors: It's about their ability to rewire trauma, break destructive cycles, and create conditions for deep healing. And this time, instead of being dismissed as mystical nonsense, the conversation is grounded in hard data, brain scans, and clinical trials.

Despite the excitement, psychedelics aren't a magic bullet. They aren't a one-size-fits-all cure, and they come with risks as well as rewards. The wrong dose, the wrong setting, or an unprepared mind can turn a promising treatment into a disaster. Some experience profound healing, while others spiral into psychosis, re-traumatization, or dissociation.

So, what do we actually know? How do these substances work? What are their real risks and benefits? And—perhaps most importantly—do they have a place in PTSD treatment?

Leading Psychedelics

LSD (Lysergic Acid Diethylamide)

LSD is the undisputed heavyweight of the psychedelic world—tiny doses can send reality into a full-blown kaleidoscopic meltdown for eight to twelve hours. Originally derived from a rye fungus (because, of course, nature had to hide mind-bending chemicals in bread mold), LSD hijacks serotonin receptors, creating intense visual distortions, deep introspection, and time dilation that can make minutes feel like centuries. Some swear by its potential to treat depression, anxiety, and PTSD, while others end up stuck in an existential horror show, convinced they've discovered the true nature of the universe...and that it hates them. It's a powerful tool, but also a wild card—making it difficult to control in clinical settings.

Pros: LSD has shown promise in enhancing neuroplasticity—the brain's ability to rewire itself—which is why some researchers believe it could be a game changer for PTSD and depression. Unlike pharmaceuticals that dull symptoms, LSD can allow people to confront and process trauma from a radically new perspective. Many users report experiencing a deep sense of interconnectedness, increased emotional openness, and a shift in long-held negative thought patterns. In controlled settings, LSD-assisted therapy has produced long-term improvements in anxiety and mood disorders with just one or two sessions, which is practically unheard of in conventional psychiatry.

Cons: The downside? Predictability—or rather, the lack of it. Even in clinical settings, there's no way to guarantee that an LSD experience will be enlightening instead of terrifying. "Bad trips" are a real risk, especially for individuals with underlying mental health conditions. And because the effects last so long, a bad trip isn't something you can simply sleep off in a couple of hours. There's also the issue of intensity—LSD doesn't just take you for a ride, it takes the steering wheel and locks the doors. While it's not physically addictive, psychological dependence is possible, particularly for those chasing its euphoric or mind-expanding effects. Plus, in the wrong hands or used irresponsibly, it can push latent psychosis to the surface, making it a high-risk option for anyone predisposed to schizophrenia or severe anxiety disorders.

Psilocybin (Magic Mushrooms)

If LSD is a rollercoaster, psilocybin is a guided nature walk—still bizarre, but often more organic and introspective. Found in certain fungi, these "magic" mushrooms have been used for centuries in spiritual ceremonies, making people feel one with the universe…or, at the very least, with their carpet, which now seems to be breathing. Psilocybin affects serotonin pathways, leading to everything from euphoria and emotional breakthroughs to full-blown hallucinations. It's currently being studied as a treatment for depression and trauma, and while the results are promising, "bad trips" can hit like a freight train, leaving users stuck in loops of paranoia or existential dread. Set and setting matter—this is not the kind of thing you want to take at a crowded music festival if you're on the verge of a breakdown.

Pros: Psilocybin has gained serious traction in the mental health world, and for good reason. Unlike traditional antidepressants that you have to take daily, a single guided psilocybin session can produce lasting improvements in depression, anxiety, and PTSD. It promotes neuroplasticity, meaning the brain literally rewires itself in ways that can help break long-standing patterns of negative thinking. Many users report feeling a profound sense of clarity, connection, and emotional release—sometimes experiencing what can only be described as a "spiritual reset." Unlike LSD, psilocybin trips tend to feel more natural, fluid, and introspective rather than overwhelming. Studies at Johns Hopkins and UCLA have shown that, when taken in a controlled setting with proper guidance, psilocybin-assisted therapy can be remarkably effective at reducing end-of-life anxiety, major depression, and even addiction.[18],[19] Best of all? It's relatively short-lived compared to LSD, typically lasting four to six hours instead of a full-day commitment to an altered reality.

Cons: Psilocybin is not a magic bullet. "Bad trips" can hit hard and fast, especially for those dealing with unresolved trauma, anxiety, or a fragile mental state. While the trip itself may be shorter than LSD, it can still feel like an eternity if you're stuck in a loop of paranoia or existential dread. And while most people return to baseline without issue, some report lingering emotional instability or a resurfacing of past trauma in the weeks after a trip. The effectiveness of psilocybin is also highly dependent on "set and setting"—a clinical, well supported environment can lead to breakthroughs, while taking it in an unpredictable or chaotic setting can be a recipe for psychological distress. While it's not considered physically addictive, some users develop a pattern of overuse,

---

18 Griffiths, R. R., Johnson, M. W., Carducci, M. A., Umbricht, A., Richards, W. A., Richards, B. D., Cosimano, M. P., & Klinedinst, M. A. (2016). Psilocybin produces substantial and sustained decreases in depression and anxiety in patients with life-threatening cancer: A randomized double-blind trial. *Journal of Psychopharmacology, 30*(12), 1181–1197. https://doi.org/10.1177/0269881116675513

19 Martinez, M. (2022, August 24). Psychedelics may lessen fear of death and dying, similar to feelings reported by those who've had near death experiences. *Johns Hopkins Medicine.* https://www.hopkinsmedicine.org/news/newsroom/news-releases/2022/08/psychedelics-may-lessen-fear-of-death-and-dying-similar-to-feelings-reported-by-those-whove-had-near-death-experiences?utm_source=chatgpt.com

chasing the insight and euphoria rather than doing the work to integrate the experience. Finally, while rare, those predisposed to schizophrenia or psychotic disorders may find that psilocybin exacerbates their condition, making it a potentially risky choice for certain individuals.

Ibogaine

Ibogaine is the black sheep of the psychedelic family—equal parts promising and terrifying. Found in the root bark of the *Tabernanthe iboga* shrub, ibogaine has been used for centuries in West African Bwiti ceremonies as a spiritual and initiatory tool. But in modern times, it has gained a reputation as a potential addiction interrupter, particularly for opioids.

Unlike traditional detox methods, which rely on slow tapering and medication-assisted treatment, ibogaine seems to reboot the brain's addiction pathways in a way that nothing else does. Users descried an intense, dreamlike state lasting up to twenty-four hours, during which they relive past traumas, confront deep emotional wounds, and—if all goes well—emerge with significantly reduced cravings and withdrawal symptoms. For some, it's a second chance at life; for others, it's a nightmarish ordeal they'd rather forget.

Veterans Exploring Treatment Solutions (VETS), in collaboration with Stanford University, has supported a pioneering study on the effects of ibogaine therapy for veterans suffering from TBI and PTSD. These efforts represent the beginning of a more rigorous scientific look at what this controversial compound may offer—not just for addiction, but for deep-rooted psychological trauma. But if you're considering this therapy, it is absolutely essential to undergo proper cardiac monitoring and be in the care of trained medical professionals who can intervene immediately if complications arise.

Pros: If there's one thing ibogaine is known for, it's breaking addiction cycles—particularly for those dependent on opioids, cocaine, or other compulsive substances. Unlike conventional rehab, where withdrawal symptoms can be excruciating and relapse is common, ibogaine can drastically reduce or even eliminate withdrawal after just one session. Some users describe waking up feeling as if their addiction was "erased," no longer controlled by the obsessive cravings that once dictated their every move. Studies in animal models support this, showing that ibogaine reduces self-administration of opioids, cocaine, and alcohol. While research on humans is still limited, the anecdotal evidence is staggering. Many who have tried everything—rehab, therapy, medication—report that ibogaine was the only thing that gave them a real chance at recovery. But its power goes beyond just stopping cravings. Ibogaine forces users into deep psychological introspection, often making them confront past traumas that contributed to their addiction in the first place. Some describe meeting "entities" or reliving painful memories in vivid detail, as if their subconscious is unraveling before them. When guided properly, this can be transformative—helping users process emotions that have been buried for years. Unlike traditional psychedelics, which focus on perception shifts and spiritual awakenings, ibogaine is more of a biological reset—hitting both the mind and the nervous system in ways we still don't fully understand.

Cons: Ibogaine is not a casual experience—it's an intense, physically taxing ordeal that can literally stop your heart. One of its most well-documented risks is QT interval prolongation, a cardiac effect that can lead to a fatal arrhythmia called torsades de pointes. Multiple deaths have been linked to ibogaine use, often due to undetected heart conditions or improper dosing. That's why reputable clinics perform extensive cardiac screening before treatment. But in underground settings—where ibogaine is often administered without medical oversight—these risks skyrocket. Medical monitoring isn't optional; it's essential. Beyond the cardiac dangers, ibogaine can cause neurological side effects like ataxia (loss of motor control), seizures, and extreme disorientation. Some users have reported lingering cognitive issues long after the experience, with cases of mania, paranoia, and hallucinogen persisting perception disorder (HPPD). And let's not forget the sheer intensity of the trip itself—many describe it as one of the most difficult, grueling experiences of their lives. This isn't a recreational drug; it's a high-stakes gamble with your mind and body.

Then there's the problem of relapse. While ibogaine can eliminate withdrawal symptoms and cravings, it doesn't magically cure addiction. Behavioral patterns, emotional wounds, and lifestyle factors still need to be addressed. Without proper aftercare, some users eventually return to drug use—leading to an even greater risk of overdose due to decreased tolerance. Ibogaine is one of the most powerful tools in addiction treatment, but it's also one of the most dangerous. For those who have exhausted every option—rehab, therapy, medication—it might be worth considering, but only in a medically supervised setting with strict screening and emergency care on standby. This isn't a miracle cure or a quick fix—it's an intense, high-risk intervention that can either break the cycle of addiction or push the body beyond its limits.

DMT (Dimethyltryptamine) and Ayahuasca

DMT is like stepping through a wormhole into another dimension, and it does it in record time—an entire trip can last just ten to fifteen minutes, but in that time, people often describe visiting alien realms, meeting strange entities, or experiencing their own death and rebirth. This "spirit molecule" is naturally found in certain plants and even the human brain, though no one quite knows why. Ayahuasca, a South American brew containing DMT, extends the experience to several hours and is used in traditional ceremonies for deep psychological and spiritual healing. Some describe ayahuasca as life-changing, others as a cosmic boot camp where Mother Nature force-feeds them their worst traumas before purging their demons (sometimes literally, in the form of violent vomiting). It's not for the faint of heart, but some research suggests it may help with PTSD and emotional healing.

Pros: DMT and ayahuasca are some of the most intense, transformative psychedelics known to humanity, and for many, that's exactly the draw. Unlike other psychedelics that gently nudge your perception, DMT kicks down the door and launches you into an entirely different reality. People report profound insights, spiritual awakenings, and encounters with what feel like divine or interdimensional beings. Ayahuasca, in particular, has been used for centuries in traditional Amazonian healing ceremonies and is now being studied for its potential to treat PTSD, depression, and addiction. Unlike traditional antidepressants, which often require daily use, a single ayahuasca experience—when done correctly in a structured, supportive setting—can lead to lasting psychological breakthroughs. Some studies suggest that it increases neuroplasticity, allowing the brain to rewire old traumas and destructive thought patterns. For those who feel stuck in their healing journey, DMT and ayahuasca offer a radical shift in perspective—one that many say has changed their lives for the better.

Cons: This is not a recreational experience. Both DMT and ayahuasca demand a level of psychological resilience that not everyone has, and for some, the experience can be terrifying. The short duration of DMT means that while the trip itself is fast, it can feel like an eternity inside the altered state—especially if it takes a dark turn. Ayahuasca, on the other hand, is a grueling multi-hour ordeal that often comes with intense nausea, vomiting, and purging, which shamans describe as a form of spiritual detox, but which (in reality) is just physically miserable. There's also the issue of control—once you take DMT, there's no dialing it back. Unlike psilocybin or LSD, where you can somewhat navigate the experience, DMT takes the wheel entirely. Additionally, those with a history of schizophrenia or psychotic disorders are at risk for serious psychological destabilization. Another major downside? The ayahuasca tourism industry is booming, and not all retreats are legitimate—some are run by opportunists looking to profit off the psychedelic renaissance, and safety is far from guaranteed. If you're considering it, make sure you're in the hands of an experienced, ethical guide.

MDMA (Ecstasy/Molly)

MDMA is the extroverted cousin of the psychedelics—less about hallucinations and more about emotional breakthroughs and intense connection. Technically an entactogen rather than a true psychedelic, MDMA floods the brain with serotonin, making people feel euphoric, open-hearted, and deeply empathetic. It's currently in phase III clinical trials as a treatment for PTSD, where it's shown incredible promise in helping patients process trauma without the overwhelming emotional pain. But there's a downside: MDMA can deplete serotonin, causing "suicide Tuesday" (that depressing crash after a weekend rave) and, at high doses, can be neurotoxic.

Pros: MDMA-assisted therapy has been making headlines for its potential to revolutionize PTSD treatment, and the results so far have been compelling. Unlike traditional talk therapy, where patients often struggle to access and process their trauma due to fear and emotional shutdown, MDMA allows them to revisit these memories without the usual fight-or-flight response. This makes it easier for therapists to guide patients through deeply buried pain in just a handful of sessions. The drug's ability to induce feelings of connection and empathy has also shown promise in repairing damaged relationships, which is why some couples have even used it to rebuild trust. Under strict clinical supervision, MDMA therapy can lead to healing—but that's the key phrase: *strict clinical supervision.*

Cons: MDMA is also one of the most dangerous drugs on this list when misused. First, there's the risk of permanent neurological damage. Unlike classic psychedelics, which primarily act on serotonin receptors without significantly depleting them, MDMA floods the brain with serotonin while also blocking its reabsorption. This can leave users emotionally drained for days, sometimes even weeks, leading to severe depressive crashes. And repeated use? That can fry the serotonin system entirely, leading to long-term emotional blunting, cognitive impairments, and anhedonia (the inability to feel pleasure). Then there's another issue—MDMA raises body temperature, which can be deadly in certain settings. In club and festival environments, people have literally cooked themselves from the inside out—overheating while dancing for hours, dehydrated, disoriented, and unable to cool down. And that's before we even touch the ethical minefield of MDMA therapy. There are stories that still haunt me—people in the '70s at makeshift retreats, overheating, delirious, and drinking from toilets just to stay alive.

This isn't just some warm, fuzzy experience where people hold hands and talk about their childhood—MDMA makes users highly suggestible and emotionally vulnerable. In controlled trials, therapists are required to follow strict protocols, but even then, there have been cases of abuse, including a high-profile scandal where a researcher sexually assaulted multiple patients under the influence. If this happens in supposedly regulated clinical settings, imagine the risks in underground or amateur "healing" circles.

Lastly, the recreational market is a Russian roulette of chemical nightmares. Street MDMA is often cut with meth, fentanyl, or other synthetic stimulants, making it unpredictable and highly dangerous. Even a single bad batch can be fatal. People assume "molly" is pure MDMA, but it's not: The reality is that most of what's sold as MDMA is a toxic mystery mix, and users often have no idea what they're actually ingesting. Bottom line? MDMA has real therapeutic potential, but its risks are severe and often downplayed by advocates. Used responsibly in a clinical setting, it may help heal trauma, but outside of that? It's a chemical minefield, and one wrong step can have permanent, life-altering consequences.

Ketamine

Ketamine doesn't play by the same rules as traditional psychedelics. Originally developed as an anesthetic (and still used in veterinary surgery—ask any horse), it induces a dissociative state where people feel detached from their body and surroundings. Unlike LSD or psilocybin, ketamine doesn't work by flooding the brain with serotonin. Instead, it targets glutamate, a neurotransmitter that plays a key role in learning, memory, and mood regulation. The result? Rapid shifts in perception and, for some, an almost immediate relief from depression—sometimes within hours. That's a game-changer in a world where conventional antidepressants take weeks to kick in, if they work at all. Already

FDA approved for treatment-resistant depression, ketamine clinics are popping up everywhere, offering hope to those who've exhausted other options. I've seen firsthand how powerful it can be in my own practice. For patients who've been stuck in a relentless cycle of trauma and despair, ketamine can open a door that nothing else has been able to budge.

Pros: Ketamine's ability to provide rapid relief from depression, PTSD, and suicidal ideation makes it one of the most promising breakthroughs in mental health treatment in decades.

Unlike traditional antidepressants, which can take weeks or even months to take effect (if they work at all), ketamine works almost immediately by increasing neuroplasticity—the brain's ability to form new connections. For those stuck in cycles of trauma, this is a game-changer. It doesn't just mask symptoms; it creates a window where the nervous system is more flexible, more open to change.

In my own practice, I've seen firsthand how powerful ketamine can be, especially when paired with the stellate ganglion block (SGB). For veterans and Special Forces operators who've spent years in high-stress environments, their nervous systems often get locked into overdrive. Ketamine, when used strategically, can help break that cycle, allowing the brain to reset and shift out of survival mode. It has also been instrumental in treating traumatic brain injury (TBI)—a condition that's notoriously difficult to address with conventional treatments. I've worked with countless warriors who have walked into treatment weighed down by years of unrelenting symptoms and walked out with a sense of clarity and relief they hadn't felt in years.

Unlike classic psychedelics like LSD or psilocybin, which require long, guided sessions, ketamine can be administered in a clinical setting without an extensive therapeutic process—though integration afterward is still key to making the effects last. It has also been used successfully in emergency psychiatric situations, particularly for those in acute suicidal crisis, making it a lifesaving tool in ways other psychedelics aren't.

Cons: Like any powerful tool, it's all about how it's used. At the right doses, in the right setting, ketamine can be transformative. But at high doses or without proper medical oversight, some people experience dissociation that can feel unsettling—often referred to as the "K-hole," where time distorts, surroundings become unfamiliar, and reality itself feels out of reach. Some find this to be a deeply introspective or even spiritual experience, while others find it disorienting. There's also been a recent surge in ketamine clinics across the country, and while many are run by responsible medical professionals, others function more like high-end IV lounges—churning patients through without much attention to long-term healing. Without proper guidance and integration, some people may find the effects short-lived, requiring repeated sessions without truly addressing the root of their trauma.

That's why in my work, I don't see ketamine as a standalone solution—it's a tool, and when combined with SGB and other nervous system-focused treatments, it becomes exponentially more effective. It's not about just feeling better for a few hours; it's about resetting the system and giving the brain the space to heal. When used correctly, it's not just relief—it's transformation.

Mescaline (Peyote and San Pedro Cactus)

Used by Indigenous cultures for thousands of years, mescaline offers a gentler, more philosophical trip compared to other psychedelics. Think of it as the wise elder of the group—it doesn't yank you into a vortex of alien dimensions but instead invites you to sit under a tree and contemplate the meaning of life. Found in cacti like peyote and San Pedro, mescaline induces vivid visual hallucinations, shifts in perception, and deep emotional processing. Unlike LSD or psilocybin, mescaline often provides a dreamlike, expansive state rather than ego death or intense dissolution. While research on its therapeutic potential is limited, Indigenous wisdom suggests it's been used for healing long before the modern world caught on.

Pros: Mescaline is often described as one of the most grounding psychedelics, providing a deep sense of introspection and connection rather than the disorienting, high-speed mind warp of LSD or DMT. Its historical use in Indigenous ceremonies speaks to its role as a tool for healing, self-discovery, and spiritual connection. Unlike shorter-acting psychedelics, the effects of mescaline unfold gradually over several hours, allowing for a more organic and immersive experience. Many users report a profound sense of clarity, emotional release, and enhanced appreciation for nature. Compared to other psychedelics, it also tends to produce fewer instances of paranoia or overwhelming fear, making it a more accessible option for those wary of intense ego dissolution. Some research suggests that mescaline may hold potential in treating depression and PTSD, though formal studies remain scarce.

Cons: While mescaline may be gentler in its psychological effects, it's not without its challenges. The trip can last ten to twelve hours, which, if things take a dark turn, can feel like an eternity. Nausea and vomiting are almost a given—many people describe the first phase of a mescaline experience as a battle with their stomach before the real journey even begins. Unlike psilocybin or MDMA, which are gaining traction in clinical settings, mescaline remains relatively under-researched, meaning its long-term effects aren't as well understood.

PCP (Phencyclidine aka Angel Dust)

PCP is the wild card of this list, and not in a good way. Originally developed as a surgical anesthetic for animals, it was abandoned when doctors realized that instead of just numbing pain, it made patients hallucinate, dissociate, and sometimes become violently aggressive. Unlike traditional psychedelics, PCP doesn't create beautiful fractal patterns or moments of spiritual clarity—it often induces paranoia, psychosis, and a complete disconnect from reality. It has a high risk of addiction, can cause severe psychological effects, and frankly, has little to no place in modern psychiatric treatment.

Pros: If you're looking for a drug that makes you feel invincible, detached from reality, and possibly willing to fight a moving car—PCP might be for you (it shouldn't be). Some users report a sense of superhuman strength and pain resistance, which might explain why it's been the subject of so many bizarre headlines. There was a time when it was studied for its anesthetic properties, and technically, it *does* numb pain—just not in any way that leads to a positive medical outcome. Unlike traditional psychedelics, which focus on perception shifts and emotional breakthroughs, PCP's main claim to fame is making people forget who they are, where they are, and why climbing a telephone pole suddenly seems like a good idea.

Cons: Where to begin? PCP has a high risk of addiction and can cause permanent neurological damage with repeated use. Unlike LSD or psilocybin, which primarily affect serotonin, PCP messes with glutamate and dopamine, which regulate pain perception, cognition, and motor function. In small doses, it can cause confusion, paranoia, and hallucinations. In higher doses, aggression, psychosis, and complete detachment from reality take over. Some users describe feeling *unstoppable,* which is all fun and games until they run headfirst through a glass window or attack first responders (both of which have actually happened).

Long-term use can lead to severe memory impairment, depression, and schizophrenia-like symptoms—even after stopping the drug. And if that wasn't enough, overdose can lead to seizures, respiratory failure, and death. Unlike ketamine, which has found a place in modern medicine, PCP is one of the few substances on this list that has zero legitimate therapeutic value. It's a neuroscientist's nightmare, a doctor's worst-case scenario, and a first responder's least favorite call. Bottom line? PCP isn't a tool for healing—it's a fast track to absolute chaos.

So, we've covered the big hitters—LSD, psilocybin, DMT, ketamine, MDMA, ibogaine, and so on. The heavyweights of the alternative therapy world. The kind of stuff that makes people see geometric patterns, confront their deepest traumas, or, in some cases, temporarily forget they have a body. If your first thought was, *"Whoa, those are a little intense,"* I don't blame you. Psychedelics are powerful tools, but not everyone wants to (or should) launch themselves into an interdimensional wormhole just to work through their emotional baggage.

Fortunately, there are other ways to support healing—ones that don't involve tripping face-first into the void. These might not be as dramatic as ibogaine rewiring your brain overnight, but they're effective in their own right. Think of them as supportive therapies—practices that work alongside other treatments to help regulate the nervous system, improve mental health, and create the conditions for lasting change.

Nondrug Related Alternative Therapies

Transcranial Magnetic Stimulation (TMS)

Transcranial magnetic stimulation (TMS) is a noninvasive treatment that uses magnetic fields to stimulate specific areas of the brain involved in mood regulation. Unlike antidepressants, which flood the entire system with chemicals, or electroconvulsive therapy (ECT), which induces seizures, TMS targets the brain directly—no surgery, no anesthesia, no systemic side effects. Originally FDA approved for treatment-resistant depression, TMS has since expanded its reach into conditions like obsessive-compulsive disorder (OCD), migraines, and even smoking cessation. And while researchers continue to explore its potential for PTSD, chronic pain, and neurological disorders, one thing is clear: TMS represents a fundamentally different way to approach mental health treatment—one that doesn't rely on swallowing a daily pill and hoping for the best.

The process itself is simple, at least in theory. During a session, an electromagnetic coil is placed against the scalp, delivering targeted magnetic pulses to stimulate the neural pathways that depression has dampened. Think of it like jump-starting a car battery—the goal is to get those circuits firing again. In some cases, patients feel relief within weeks, something unheard of in the world of conventional antidepressants, which can take months to show results—if they work at all. But like any treatment that promises a breakthrough, TMS isn't perfect. It requires a serious time commitment, it's not cheap, and while many patients experience relief, others feel nothing at all. So, is it a revolutionary tool for healing, or just another expensive gamble? Let's break it down.

Pros: For those who have tried every antidepressant on the market and walked out of more therapy sessions than they can count, TMS can be a lifeline. Unlike medication, which floods the body with chemicals and causes a laundry list of unwanted side effects, TMS only affects the targeted brain regions, leaving the rest of the body alone. That means no weight gain, no sexual dysfunction, no emotional numbing—just direct stimulation to the areas of the brain that need it.

Another major win? It doesn't require surgery or anesthesia. Unlike deep brain stimulation, which involves implanting electrodes, TMS is completely noninvasive. Patients come in, sit down, get their treatment, and leave—no recovery time, no hospital stay, no major disruption to their lives.

Perhaps the biggest selling point is that it works when nothing else does. For people battling treatment-resistant depression, where traditional methods have failed, TMS has been a game changer. Studies show that 50 to 60 percent of these patients experience significant symptom relief, and about 30 percent achieve full remission. That might not sound like a cure-all, but in the mental health world, those are impressive numbers. And unlike ECT, which can cause severe memory loss, TMS leaves cognitive function intact. In fact, some patients even report feeling sharper and more focused after treatment.

Cons: For all its benefits, TMS is not an easy fix. First, there's the time commitment. A full course of treatment means daily sessions, five days a week, for four to six weeks. Each session lasts twenty to forty minutes, which might not seem like much—until you realize you're committing to weeks of your life sitting in a chair while a machine taps away at your skull. For anyone with a packed schedule, that's a serious hurdle. Side effects, while generally mild, aren't nonexistent. The most common complaints include scalp discomfort, headaches, and facial muscle twitching during treatment. These are minor annoyances for most, but for a small percentage of patients, TMS can trigger migraines or worsen existing headaches. And then there are the rare but serious risks. Seizures, while extremely uncommon, can happen—especially in individuals with a history of epilepsy. People with bipolar disorder also need to be cautious, as TMS can trigger manic episodes. Finally, there's the biggest drawback of all: It doesn't work for everyone. About 40 to

50 percent of patients don't see a meaningful improvement, which, after spending weeks and thousands of dollars on treatment, can feel like a crushing disappointment.

Animal-Assisted Therapy: Because Sometimes, Dogs Are Better Than People

If you've ever had a bad day and been instantly comforted by a dog, congratulations—you've already experienced a form of animal therapy. The concept is simple: animals make humans feel better. Their presence has been shown to lower blood pressure, reduce cortisol (the stress hormone), and increase oxytocin (the bonding hormone). And, unlike humans, animals don't judge, interrupt, or suggest you should "just get over it."

Animal-assisted therapy isn't just about petting a golden retriever (though that's pretty great): It's used in PTSD treatment, particularly for veterans and first responders, to help regulate the nervous system. Service dogs can be trained to recognize panic attacks before they happen, provide grounding in moments of dissociation, and even wake people from nightmares. Horses, through equine therapy, offer a unique form of biofeedback—forcing individuals to regulate their emotions, as horses pick up on subtle changes in body language and energy.

There's also something profoundly healing about simply caring for another being. For people struggling with trauma, addiction, or depression, reconnecting with an animal can be the first step toward reconnecting with themselves.

Meditation: The Ancient Art of Not Freaking Out

Meditation has been around for thousands of years, and for good reason—it works. It's essentially the opposite of the chaotic overstimulation that fuels trauma responses. Instead of reacting to stress, meditation teaches you to observe it, regulate it, and (eventually) let it go.

For people recovering from trauma, meditation helps train the nervous system to step out of fight-or-flight mode. Studies show that regular meditation shrinks the amygdala (the brain's fear center) and strengthens the prefrontal cortex (the rational part of the brain). In other words, it helps shift people from a state of survival to a state of control.

Of course, if you tell someone with PTSD to "just sit quietly and clear their mind," they might look at you like you just asked them to solve quantum physics in their sleep. That's why structured meditation techniques, like mindfulness-based stress reduction (MBSR) or guided breathwork, are often more effective than simply sitting in silence and hoping for enlightenment. It's not a magic bullet, but it's a foundational practice that, when done consistently, rewires the brain for resilience.

Hiking and Outdoor Therapy: Because Nature Doesn't Gaslight You

If there's one thing we know for sure, it's that humans weren't meant to spend all day staring at screens under fluorescent lights. We evolved to be in nature, and our nervous systems still crave it. That's why hiking, wilderness therapy, and even just spending more time outside can have profound mental health benefits. When you walk through a forest, sit by a river, or climb a mountain, your body naturally shifts into a parasympathetic (rest and recover) state. The brain gets flooded with endorphins, cortisol levels drop, and problems that felt overwhelming in a cubicle suddenly seem a little more manageable. Plus, there's something deeply symbolic about physically moving forward—step-by-step—especially for people working through trauma.

Wilderness therapy has been used with veterans, at-risk youth, and individuals struggling with addiction, and the results are undeniable. It's not just about fresh air—it's about getting out of stagnant environments, reconnecting with a primal part of yourself, and proving (to yourself) that you can keep moving forward.

What's Next: Finding the Right Path for You

By now, we've covered a lot—traditional treatments, alternative therapies, and the cutting edge options that are challenging everything we thought we knew about trauma recovery. If there's one thing that should be clear by now, it's this: there is no one-size-fits-all solution. Healing isn't about picking the most popular therapy or the one with the flashiest headlines: It's about finding what works for you—what fits your mind, your body, and your life. And that's exactly what we'll get into next. Think of this as your no BS guide to making sense of it all—one that cuts through the noise, sidesteps the hype, and helps you make informed, strategic decisions. This isn't about selling you on one treatment over another, and it's definitely not about handing you a magic cure wrapped in a bow. It's about clarity and giving you the tools to navigate this maze with confidence.

Because at the end of the day, this isn't about industry debates, clinical jargon, or what someone on the internet swears changed their life—it's about reclaiming yours. So, let's figure out your next steps—together.

CHAPTER 12

YOUR ROADMAP TO HEALING AND RECOVERY

By now, it's safe to say we've covered a lot. We've taken a deep dive into the conventional, the alternative, and the downright unorthodox when it comes to healing trauma, depression, and the nervous system. We've looked at the best and worst of pharmaceuticals, the potential of psychedelics, the precision of SGB, the rewiring effects of TMS, the dissociative magic of ketamine, and even the power of holistic approaches.

But here's the thing—knowledge is useless without action.

So now comes the real question: What do you actually *do* with all this information? How do you take everything we've talked about—therapy, medications, psychedelics, interventional treatments, holistic care—and turn it into something that actually helps you or your loved one heal? Because the last thing I want is for this book to just be another overwhelming fire hose of information. If all you walk away with is *more* to think about but no idea how to move forward, then I've failed you. And that's not happening.

I want to give you a framework, a way to cut through the noise and create a plan that's tailored to *you*. Because healing isn't about randomly throwing treatments at the wall and hoping something sticks. It's about strategy—understanding where you are, what your body needs, and what steps will actually move the needle for you. At this point, you're probably asking yourself: *How do I make smart, strategic decisions about my healing? How do I combine and sequence treatments to get the absolute best results? How do I know if trying a high-risk treatment is worth it?*

These are the questions that matter. Because the truth is, no one wants to waste their time, money, or energy on something that won't actually help. And no one wants to take unnecessary risks with their body or mind. So, in this chapter, we're going to get practical. I'll walk you through a step-by-step approach to understanding what your body needs, how to prioritize different treatments, and how to weigh the risks and rewards of each option. And by the time we're done, you'll have a clear roadmap for making decisions that serve *you.*

The Doorway Framework

There's a framework I often give people to help them understand the process of healing from trauma and I want to share it with you. When you've been carrying the weight of trauma for years, you begin to feel disconnected from your life, and before you know it, you feel like an outsider. Trauma turns you into a window gazer—a spectator to your own life. It's like you're standing outside in the cold, looking through the glass at the life you're supposed to be living. You see people laughing around the dinner table, forming deep relationships, chasing their dreams—while you're stuck on the outside, watching. You can see it all so clearly, but no matter what you do, you can't seem to step inside.

You might be physically present, but emotionally, mentally? You're standing on the other side of the glass. Conversations feel scripted, like you're just saying the right words rather than actually feeling them. You go through the motions—showing up, responding when people talk to you, even smiling at the right moments—but it's all distant, like you're watching a movie of someone else's life instead of living your own. You can feel the warmth in the room, hear the laughter, see the way people connect, but it doesn't *reach* you. It doesn't land.

Loneliness takes on a different shape here—it's not about being physically alone, it's about being unseen. It's about standing in the middle of a crowded room and feeling miles away from everyone. It's knowing you *should* feel close to the people who love you, but instead, everything is muted, dulled, happening behind glass. And the worst part? No one else knows you feel this way. From the outside, you look fine. You function. You blend in. Maybe you've even convinced yourself that this is *good enough.* That you're managing. That this is just how life is now.

So, you do what anyone would do in that situation: you push harder. You tell yourself to *snap out of it.* You force yourself into social situations that drain you. You read all the self-help books, repeat the affirmations, try to "just move on." Maybe you even get mad at yourself for still feeling this way—after all, the past is *over,* right? Shouldn't you be over it too? But that's not how trauma works. You can't break the window. No amount of willpower, self-discipline, or sheer determination is going to let you punch your way through. And the harder you try, the more frustrating it becomes. Because the problem isn't that you aren't trying hard enough—the problem is that you're trying to get inside the wrong way. What you need isn't more force. You need to find the door.

Finding the Door: The First Step to True Healing

The breakthrough comes when you realize that healing isn't about brute force—it's about strategy. Instead of throwing yourself against the window over and over, you step back, take a breath, and start looking for the door. And that begins with recognizing something most people never do: your trauma responses are not personal failings. The anxiety that grips you out of nowhere. The emotional numbness that makes everything feel distant. The hypervigilance that keeps you scanning every room for a threat that isn't there. The self-sabotage that wrecks your own happiness before someone else can take it from you.

These aren't signs that you're weak—they're survival adaptations. Your nervous system isn't broken, it's been doing exactly what it needed to do to protect you. When things went wrong—when life became unpredictable, when people who should have been safe weren't, when the world around you felt like a battlefield—your body adjusted. It shut down parts of you that were too vulnerable, kept you alert to danger, and made sure you could endure. That realization alone is a key. You are not the problem. The problem is the survival patterns you're still living by.

Finding the door means getting brutally honest with yourself—not in some vague, abstract way, but in a real, tangible, look-at-your-life-and-call-it-what-it-is kind of way. It's easy to say, "I'm fine," or "I've moved on," but if you keep ending up in the same cycles, if you feel stuck in patterns you can't seem to break, it's time to take a closer look.

A good place to start? Take a PCL-5 test—a short, evidence-based questionnaire used to screen for PTSD symptoms. Better yet, ask your spouse or someone close to you. Because here's the wild truth: nearly 50 percent of people with PTSD don't think they have it.

(*And no—denial isn't just a river in Egypt. It's a full-time residence for a lot of us.*)

- Where is life not working for you? What areas feel like a constant uphill battle, no matter how hard you try?
- What are the symptoms of your trauma showing up as? Is it the relationships that never seem to work out? The exhaustion that never goes away. The constant background hum of anxiety or numbness that makes everything feel distant.
- Where do you keep making excuses for things that aren't okay? Do you tell yourself you're just bad at relationships when, really, you're terrified of letting someone get too close? Do you dismiss your burnout as "just the way life is" instead of recognizing you're running on empty because you never learned to feel safe when you slow down?
- What are the patterns you keep repeating? The friendships that end the same way, the moments where you sabotage yourself right before something good happens, the ways you shut down when you should speak up?

- Where are you fooling yourself? Where have you convinced yourself that "it's not that bad" when deep down, you know it is?

This isn't about judgment—it's about clarity. Because if you can't see the patterns, you can't break them. And if you keep telling yourself a story that doesn't match reality, you'll keep living inside that same story, stuck in the same loop. Healing starts with awareness. Not fixing, not forcing, just noticing. Taking inventory. Calling things what they are. That's how you stop pressing your face against the glass and start looking for the door.

And here's the thing—this stage isn't about fixing yourself.

That's not the goal. Not yet. This is about *understanding* yourself. Because you can't break a cycle if you don't know you're in one. You can't move forward if you don't know what's been holding you back. And you sure can't heal if you're still blaming yourself for the ways your body and mind tried to keep you alive. This is where you step away from the window and admit that just watching life from the outside isn't enough anymore. You're done pressing your face against the glass. Done wishing things were different while repeating the same patterns that keep you stuck. You're ready to step inside. And that means it's time to find the *keys.*

Choosing the Right Keys: Unlocking Your Healing in the Right Order

So, you've found the door. That's a massive first step. But here's the frustrating part—you can't just waltz through it because the darn thing is locked. And not just with a single deadbolt, but with multiple locks, layered on top of each other like some kind of trauma-fortified security system. And now, here you are, standing at the threshold, holding a *jangling* keyring of potential interventions. Therapy. Medication. Psychedelics. TMS. SGB. Breathwork. Nutrition. Which one do you use? Which one actually works?

The truth? Not every key fits every lock. Healing isn't a one-size-fits-all journey, and throwing random treatments at yourself without a plan is like trying to crack a safe by mindlessly spinning the dial and hoping something clicks. Some keys won't work at all. Some only work if used in a specific order. And others? They might only turn halfway before getting stuck—because they're not enough on their own. So, how do you choose? How do you make sure you're using the right key at the right time, instead of wasting energy on something that won't budge the lock?

You start with strategy.

1. Check Your Baseline Keys First

Before jumping into advanced treatments, you need to make sure you've checked on all your body's basic functions. Think of it like trying to build a house—you wouldn't start with the roof, right? You'd lay the groundwork first. If your system is running on empty—chronically sleep-deprived, undernourished, and constantly inflamed—then no fancy intervention is going to stick. Your body needs a solid baseline before it can handle deeper healing.

- **Sleep**—If you're running on fumes, healing is infinitely harder. Quality sleep isn't a luxury—it's a biological requirement for nervous system repair.
- **Nutrition**—Your brain is an organ. It needs fuel. If your body is inflamed or deficient in key nutrients, your nervous system stays stuck in survival mode.
- **Movement**—Trauma lives in the body. Strength training, yoga, walking—whatever gets you moving—isn't optional, it's medicine.
- **Mindfulness and Breathwork**—If you can't regulate your breath, you can't regulate your nervous system. Breath is the fast-track to shifting out of fight-or-flight.
- **Hormones**—Imbalanced hormones (like cortisol, testosterone, or estrogen) can hijack your mental health. You can't outtalk a hormone crash.

- **Thyroid**—A sluggish thyroid mimics depression and anxiety. If your energy is shot and your mood's in the tank, it's worth checking.
- **Heavy Metals and Toxins**—Environmental toxins can quietly sabotage your healing. High levels of heavy metals like lead or mercury can dysregulate your brain, gut, and immune system.

It's worth doing comprehensive lab work to get a clear picture of what's going on under the hood—testing your hormone levels, thyroid function, nutrient status, and toxin load can reveal hidden obstacles that might be quietly sabotaging your healing.

2. The Therapeutic Keys

If trauma has hijacked your nervous system—leaving you stuck in fight, flight, freeze, or shut down—then you need tools to bring your system back to balance. These keys don't process trauma directly; instead, they create the conditions that allow healing to happen by regulating your physiology. Think of them as stabilizing the storm before you start rebuilding.

- **Breathwork and HRV Training**—These practices help rewire your body's ability to return to a calm state instead of staying in high alert mode. Heart rate variability (HRV) is a measure of how adaptable your nervous system is—higher HRV means your body can shift gears more easily. Breathwork and vagus nerve stimulation improve HRV, slow the heart rate, and signal safety to the brain.
- **Somatic Experiencing and Trauma-Informed Yoga**—Trauma isn't just in your head—it lives in your body. These body-based approaches help you reconnect with physical sensations, release stored tension, and reestablish a sense of safety in your own skin. They help you move from dissociation to embodiment, one breath and stretch at a time.

- **Psychotherapy**—When your system is regulated enough to engage, talk therapy can be incredibly powerful. It provides a structured space to process emotions, identify harmful patterns, and develop healthier coping strategies. When paired with physiological support, therapy becomes not just tolerable—but transformational.

3. The Recalibration Keys

For some people, the Baseline Keys and Therapeutic Keys are enough to get back on track. With the right combination of movement, nutrition, breathwork, and therapy, their system finds balance again, and healing begins to unfold.

But for others, it's not enough. No amount of breathwork, therapy, or superfood salads can pull them out of the danger loop—the locked-in survival state where their nervous system refuses to shift. They're stuck, no matter how much insight they gain or how hard they try. Their system isn't resisting out of stubbornness—it's trapped. And that's when deeper interventions become not just helpful, but necessary. This is where Recalibration Keys come in. These aren't about gradual progress or mindset shifts—these are interventions designed to reset the system at a foundational level so that real healing can begin. Only when the system is recalibrated can deep transformation happen—where old patterns get rewired, and survival-based responses start to loosen their grip.

- **SGB (Stellate Ganglion Block)**—This is like a physiological reset button for an overactive fight-or-flight response. It won't process trauma for you, but it can make your nervous system quiet enough to finally do the work.
- **Neurofeedback and TMS**—Trauma physically changes your brain. With enough treatments, TMS can help retrain and reset brain patterns that have been altered by chronic stress and PTSD/PTSI.

For many people, this is the stage where therapy actually works, because your system is finally regulated enough to engage with it.

4. *The Breakthrough Keys*

For those with severe, complex, or treatment-resistant trauma—what some might call "big f--cking trauma"—standard approaches might only get you so far. But let's be clear: it's not the size of the event that earns that label, it's how your specific body responded to it. Trauma isn't a competition. Yet people constantly judge themselves—measuring their pain against someone else's war stories like it's some kind of trauma Olympics. You see someone flexing their BFT muscles and think, "Well, I haven't been through *that,* so what's wrong with me?"

The truth? Your nervous system decides; not your ego, and not the headlines. If your system is stuck—if you're locked in survival mode and nothing's working—it doesn't matter what caused it. You don't need to win the "worst story" award to deserve real help. Sometimes, your body needs a stronger nudge to break free.

That's where the Breakthrough Keys come in:

- **Ketamine Therapy**—Fast-acting, legally available in many clinics, ketamine can create rapid shifts in mood and perception. It's often used to break cycles of depression and unstick the brain from rigid, looping thought patterns. This may potentially help with suicidal tendencies.
- **Psychedelic-Assisted Therapy (MDMA, Psilocybin, Ayahuasca, Ibogaine)**—These aren't magic bullets. But when done correctly, in the right setting with the right support, they can break through deeply embedded trauma, giving access to parts of the self that traditional methods can't reach.
- **Immersion Retreats and Intensive Therapy Programs**—Sometimes you need a full system reboot. These retreats create a safe, focused container for deep work, away from distractions, triggers, and day-to-day stressors. They're designed for people who feel stuck and need an intensive push toward healing.

The biggest mistake people make in healing? They quit too soon. Don't: If you haven't found what works for you yet, it doesn't mean you're broken, it just means you haven't found the right key—*yet.* Many people try one or two things, don't see results fast enough, and assume nothing will work. But healing is a *process,* not a single event. It requires patience, trial and error, and sometimes multiple keys used in the right sequence before the locks finally release. Consider treatments that are easy to comply with—low-risk, low-barrier options that gently signal safety to your nervous system. These interventions don't demand your deepest emotional labor on day one. They're about building momentum, stabilizing your foundation, and preparing your system to respond to deeper work. If one key doesn't work, it doesn't mean healing isn't possible; it means you might need a different key—or a different order. So don't give up: The door is there, and the locks *can* be opened. And the life waiting on the other side? It's worth fighting for.

Opening the Door: The Breakthrough Moment

Finally, you hear it—that click. The unmistakable signal that something is different this time. The locks release. The hinges creak. And for the first time, light spills through the widening gap. This is the moment. The shift. The thing you weren't sure was possible. For some, it comes as an unmistakable wave—like the weight you've carried for years has suddenly lifted, like your body finally exhaled a breath you didn't even realize you were holding. Maybe your mind feels clearer, quieter. Maybe, for the first time in as long as you can remember, you sleep through the night without waking up in a panic. Maybe you sit down with your family, and instead of just existing in the same space, you actually *feel* present with them. It's a strange feeling at first—like stepping into a warm room after being out in the cold for so long that you forgot what warmth even felt like.

For others, it's more subtle. So subtle, in fact, that they don't even notice it at first. The shift isn't dramatic or immediate—it's quiet, steady, like a fog lifting one layer at a time. And often, it's the people around them who notice the change first. That's why I always say, *"When in doubt, ask your spouse."* They're usually the first to see the light coming back into your eyes, the tension starting to ease, the space between reaction and response growing just wide enough to breathe.

"You seem different."

"Lighter."

"Like yourself again."

At first, you might not believe them. Trauma has a way of making you doubt good things. You're used to hypervigilance, to waiting for the other shoe to drop. Feeling good—even just *okay*—can almost feel suspicious, like a setup for disappointment. But then you catch yourself laughing—*really* laughing. Or feeling safe in a way that doesn't feel like a fluke. And slowly, it sinks in: *You're inside now.* For so long, you stood outside looking in. You pressed your face against the glass, watching life happen on the other side. Now, you're here. You've stepped through the door.

And that changes everything. This moment is precious. But it's also delicate. A breakthrough is like the first flame of a fire—it needs space, air, and protection. It's a turning point, but not an endpoint. And if you're not careful, it's easy to let it slip through your fingers, to get pulled back into old ways of thinking, old environments, old cycles. Because while stepping through the door is a powerful shift, it doesn't erase the past. The habits, the defenses, the survival strategies that once kept you safe? They don't just disappear. They don't know you've found a new way. That's why what happens *next* matters just as much as the breakthrough itself.

Be selective about who you let into your space. Not everyone deserves access to this version of you. Some people—intentionally or not—thrived when you were hurting, when your boundaries were weak, when your identity was wrapped in pain. Some relationships were built on your dysfunction, and your healing threatens the foundation they stood on. That's not your burden to carry. This is a season for alignment—for surrounding yourself with people who see your growth, support your evolution, and speak to the future you're building, not the past you've outgrown. And that means being willing to remove toxic people from your life. Protect your peace. Guard your energy. You're not just healing—you're becoming. Not everyone gets to come with you.

Refuse stressors that could derail your progress. You don't need to fight unnecessary battles right now. Avoid drama, conflict, and anything that tries to drag you back into survival mode. Your nervous system is recalibrating—don't throw it back into chaos. Even small stressors can shake a fragile breakthrough, and right now, your job is to protect what's growing inside you.

Allow yourself to hope. I know, hope is risky. It feels vulnerable, especially if you've been disappointed before. But this moment? This shift? It's real. And it's something you can build on. Let yourself believe, even just a little, that things can get better. That you don't have to keep living in the patterns of the past. That maybe, just maybe, this time is different.

Because this isn't the end of the story. In fact, this is just the beginning.

Walking the Path: Making Healing Your New Normal

Once the door is open, *this* is where the magic happens. Not because you're done (far from it) but because you now have something you didn't have before: a real shot at building the life you want. This is where people go wrong. They mistake a breakthrough for a cure. They assume that just because they *feel* different—lighter, clearer, more present—that the work is done. But the truth is, breakthroughs don't fix everything. *They create an opportunity.*

Think of it like clearing a path in the wilderness. Before, you were lost in a tangled mess of branches, stumbling through the dark. Now, the path is open—but you still have to *walk it.* You still have to put one foot in front of the other, making choices every day that reinforce the progress you've made. And here's the most exciting part: If you do, healing starts to snowball.

That breakthrough you had? It wasn't a onetime miracle. It was the start of a *cascade*—a ripple effect that, if nurtured, will touch every part of your life. Your body, your mind, your relationships, your energy levels, your ability to feel *fully alive.* This is where you start rebuilding, not just recovering. You're not just trying to undo damage anymore—you're creating something *better* than what was there before. A new way of being. A new normal.

Rebuilding From the Inside Out

Your breakthrough gave you an opening. Now, it's time to seize it. Because if you don't, your old habits, patterns, and physiology will pull you right back to where you started. This is the moment to go all in—to focus on every part of your body and mind that trauma has impacted so you can truly recover, rebuild, and reclaim your life. Trauma doesn't just sit in your head: it rewires your body—your hormones, your metabolism, your immune system, your gut, your sleep cycles. It dictates your cravings, your habits, your energy levels. And until you take control of those areas, your healing will always feel like an uphill battle. This is your chance to reset everything. And once you do? Your body and mind will start working *with* you instead of against you.

Your Body Can Finally Recover—But Only If You Support It

For years, your body has been in survival mode. High stress, poor sleep, erratic energy, chronic tension—it's all been part of the trauma response. And even though you may feel mentally different after your breakthrough, your body needs time to catch up. Now is the time to heal from the inside out. Your energy levels can finally return—*if you fuel your body properly.* Your digestion will improve—*if you stop feeding it junk.* Your hormones will rebalance—*but only if you prioritize recovery.* You will feel stronger—*but only if you move.*

Your body is finally in a place where it can heal—but healing isn't passive. You have to give your body the right conditions to fully repair itself. Trauma took a toll on more than just your mind; it disrupted core systems that are essential for long-term health. If you don't address these, you'll always feel like you're taking two steps forward and one step back. This isn't about chasing perfection. It's about identifying the areas that have been hit the hardest and bringing them back online so your energy, resilience, and well-being become sustainable.

1. Nutrition: Food is Medicine, Not Just Fuel

For years, your body has been running on stress hormones, not real energy. And if your diet has been full of processed, inflammatory, or nutrient-poor foods, your system is malnourished in ways that go far beyond calories.

Trauma often leads to:

- **Blood sugar instability**—Chronic stress wrecks insulin sensitivity, leading to energy crashes, mood swings, and sugar cravings.
- **Nutrient depletion**—High stress depletes key vitamins and minerals like magnesium, zinc, and B vitamins.
- **Inflammation**—Processed foods, alcohol, and sugar increase systemic inflammation, which can keep the nervous system in a heightened state.

How to fix it:

- **Prioritize whole, nutrient-dense foods.** Focus on proteins, healthy fats, fiber, and slow-digesting carbs.
- **Skip the energy drinks.** Too much caffeine spikes cortisol and crashes your nervous system.
- **Balance blood sugar.** Eat protein and fat with every meal to avoid spikes and crashes.
- **Reduce inflammatory foods.** Cut out excessive sugar, processed oils, and refined carbs.
- **Hydrate properly.** Dehydration alone can trigger stress responses.

This isn't about losing weight or chasing a fad diet—it's about fueling a body that is actively repairing itself.

2. Checking Your Hormonal Health: Trauma Leaves an Imprint

Chronic stress throws everything off balance—especially your hormones. Your body has spent years prioritizing stress hormones (cortisol and adrenaline) over everything else. That means:

- **Testosterone and estrogen levels drop**—leading to fatigue, brain fog, low motivation, and even depression.
- **Thyroid function slows down**—making weight management, energy, and metabolism a struggle.
- **Cortisol dysregulation**—leaving you wired at night and exhausted during the day.
- **Sex hormones suffer**—libido, fertility, and menstrual cycles are all affected.

What to do:

- **Get your hormones tested.** A simple blood test can tell you where you stand.
- **Support your adrenal glands.** Adaptogens like ashwagandha and rhodiola can help regulate stress hormones.
- **Prioritize sleep and recovery.** Hormones cannot rebalance if you're constantly in overdrive.
- **Consider targeted supplements.** Magnesium, zinc, vitamin D, and omega-3s all play key roles in hormonal balance.

If you ignore hormones, you'll constantly feel like you're fighting against your own body. Get them optimized, and everything gets easier.

3. Gut Health: The Brain-Gut Connection is Real

Your gut isn't just about digestion—it's a second brain. In fact, 90 percent of serotonin (your feel-good neurotransmitter) is produced in the gut. If your gut is off, your mood, energy, and focus will be too.

Trauma can lead to:

- **Dysbiosis**—An imbalance of good and bad bacteria, which affects mood and immunity.
- **Leaky gut**—Stress weakens the gut lining, allowing inflammation to spread throughout the body.
- **Slow digestion**—When your nervous system is in survival mode, digestion isn't a priority. That means bloating, discomfort, and nutrient malabsorption.

What to do:

- **Cut out gut irritants.** Gluten, excessive dairy, and processed foods can cause gut inflammation.
- **Eat fermented foods or take a probiotic.** Sauerkraut, kimchi, and kefir support a healthy microbiome.
- **Manage stress.** Your gut can't heal if you're constantly in fight-or-flight mode.
- **Support digestion.** Bitter foods, digestive enzymes, and fiber can help things move properly.

If your gut is in bad shape, your brain will feel foggy, sluggish, and off no matter what else you do.

4. Adrenal Recovery: Getting Out of Survival Mode

Your adrenal glands (the tiny glands sitting on top of your kidneys) have been on overdrive for years. They're responsible for pumping out stress hormones, and after prolonged trauma, they can either burn out completely or stay stuck in a dysfunctional cycle.

Signs your adrenals need help:

- You feel wired but tired—exhausted but can't relax.
- You rely on caffeine to function.
- You get an energy crash every afternoon.
- You struggle with motivation and focus.

What to do:

- **Reduce stimulants.** If you're relying on coffee just to get through the day, your adrenals need a break.
- **Cycle between work and recovery.** Your body isn't designed for nonstop stress. Build in true rest periods.
- **Eat balanced meals with protein and fat.** Skipping meals or eating high-carb foods can spike and crash blood sugar, making adrenal issues worse.
- **Use adaptogens.** Herbs like ashwagandha, Cordyceps, and holy basil can help regulate adrenal function.
- **Optimize sleep.** No amount of supplements can replace the recovery power of deep, quality sleep.

When your adrenals recover, your entire system stabilizes. Energy, sleep, and mood all improve.

5. Blood Sugar Stability: The Key to Consistent Energy and Mood

If your blood sugar is out of whack, you'll constantly feel anxious, irritable, fatigued, and unfocused. Trauma makes blood sugar regulation worse by increasing insulin resistance, which means energy crashes, brain fog, and constant hunger.

What to do:

- **Start the day with protein and fat.** Ditch the high-carb breakfast. Scrambled eggs with avocado will serve you better than a bagel.
- **Eat balanced meals.** Protein, healthy fats, fiber, and slow-digesting carbs keep blood sugar steady.
- **Get enough magnesium.** It's crucial for insulin regulation.
- **Move after meals.** A short walk helps keep blood sugar stable. Fix your blood sugar, and you'll experience more consistent energy, better focus, and fewer mood swings.

6. Nervous System Regulation: Your Body Needs to Feel Safe

Physical health and nervous system health go hand in hand. If your body still perceives stress as a constant threat, it won't prioritize deep healing.

What to do:

- **Get morning sunlight.** This helps regulate your circadian rhythm and stress response.
- **Grounding techniques.** Walk barefoot on the earth, sit in nature, and get real sunlight exposure.
- **Cold exposure.** Cold showers or ice baths can help retrain your stress response.
- **Deep breathing exercises.** Activates the parasympathetic nervous system, bringing calm and balance.

When your body feels safe, it shifts from surviving to thriving.

7. Your Mind Needs Stability—So You Have to Reinforce It

A breakthrough gives you clarity. But clarity fades if you don't lock it in with action. You need to create mental stability so your brain doesn't revert back to old patterns.

> **Psychotherapy isn't just for crisis—it's for reinforcement.** If you've found a therapist or healing practice that works, stick with it. Now is not the time to assume you're "fine" and drop the work. Keep unpacking, keep processing, keep expanding.
>
> **Meditation rewires your brain—but only if you do it consistently.** Even five minutes a day can strengthen the pathways in your brain that regulate emotions and stress. This is mental training, and it compounds over time.
>
> **Journaling isn't just writing—it's pattern recognition.** What's working? What's triggering? What feels different? Write it down. If you track your own patterns, you can adjust in real time instead of spiraling when things feel off.
>
> **Reduce your digital overload.** Social media, endless news cycles, mindless scrolling—it's overstimulating, addictive, and terrible for your focus. Start protecting your mental energy.

Your brain is healing. Give it the space and the tools to do it properly.

8. Sleep Is the Ultimate Reset—So Stop Treating It Like an Afterthought

Trauma wrecks sleep. High cortisol keeps you wired, hypervigilant, and restless. Poor sleep, in turn, worsens anxiety, depression, and emotional regulation. It's a vicious cycle—and now's the time to break it.

> **Set a sleep schedule and stick to it.** Go to bed and wake up at the same time every day—even on weekends. Your body craves rhythm.
>
> **Cut out blue light before bed.** Screens suppress melatonin and keep your brain wired. At least an hour before sleep, turn off the phone, dim the lights, and let your brain wind down.
>
> **Control your environment.** Make your bedroom dark, cool, and quiet. Your body is wired to sleep best in cave-like conditions.
>
> **Supplement wisely.** Magnesium, glycine, and theanine—certain natural compounds can help your nervous system relax without pharmaceuticals.
>
> **Start winding down early.** Stop trying to go from full speed stimulation to immediate sleep. Read, journal, meditate—give your brain permission to shift gears.

Good sleep is nonnegotiable for healing. Treat it that way.

Your Lifestyle Will Dictate Whether You Stay Inside or Drift Back Out

This is where healing turns into a way of life. Because at the end of the day, your lifestyle determines whether you stay inside the house or slip back into old patterns.

Choose an environment that reinforces progress. If your daily surroundings are chaotic, toxic, or full of old triggers, it will pull you back. Find a place that supports growth—physically and emotionally. Be ruthless about your relationships. Some people are good for your healing; some people aren't. Protect your energy. If someone drags you into old habits, doubt, or dysfunction, create space. Replace old coping mechanisms with better ones. The behaviors that helped you survive trauma won't help you thrive. If you're still drinking, numbing out, avoiding, procrastinating—replace those habits with something that actually serves you.

Set goals that excite you. Growth needs *direction.* If you don't give your mind something compelling to work toward, it will drift back to old patterns. Find something that challenges you, excites you, pulls you forward.

The key is momentum. When healing becomes a lifestyle, you don't have to rely on willpower—you just *become* the kind of person who naturally does the things that keep them strong.

Rebuilding Takes Strategy—But It's Worth It

Every one of these areas plays a role in how well you sustain healing. If you ignore them, progress will feel like two steps forward, one step back. But if you strategically rebuild these systems, your energy, mood, and overall well-being will snowball in the right direction. This isn't about doing everything perfectly; it's about making intentional choices that support the new life you're stepping into. Your body is ready to heal. Now, give it what it needs. You didn't do all this work to visit a better life—you did it to *live there.*

That means making a conscious choice every day to protect, reinforce, and build on the progress you've made.

- **Prioritize your health.** Your body is the launchpad for everything—your energy, your clarity, your ability to show up.

- **Sharpen your mind.** Your thoughts shape your choices, and your choices shape your life. A powerful life starts with a disciplined mind.
- **Choose your people wisely.** The right circle elevates you. The wrong one erodes you. Environment isn't neutral—it's identity in the making.
- **Live with intention.** Drift is the default. Direction is a decision. Don't wake up one day wondering how you got somewhere you never meant to go.
- **Stay consistent.** It's not the big, dramatic efforts—it's the quiet, repeated ones that rebuild you. Habits, not hype, create transformation.
- **Build momentum.** Every win fuels the next. Stack them. Let progress become your addiction.
- **Guard your energy.** Old patterns, toxic people, draining places—know what pulls you off course. Set boundaries like your future depends on it—because it does.
- **Get excited.** Healing isn't just the absence of pain—it's the presence of possibility. This is about who you're becoming. And that's worth everything.

Healing isn't about chasing breakthroughs—it's about what you do *after* the breakthrough. It's about stepping fully into the life that trauma once kept out of reach and making sure you don't just pop in for a visit—you stay. You build something real. You make it your new normal. Because that's the goal: not just to feel better for a moment, but to create a life where you're thriving in every sense.

That means treating healing like a full-body process. It's not just about your mind—it's about restoring every system that trauma disrupted. It's about fueling your body with real nutrition, checking in on your hormones, healing your gut, and rebuilding your energy from the inside out. It's about breaking old habits that kept you stuck and replacing them with ones that actually support who you're becoming. It's about choosing *who* and *what* you allow into your life—because the environment you create will either reinforce your healing or sabotage it.

Most importantly, stay consistent and be patient with yourself. Progress doesn't come from doing everything perfectly—it comes from showing up, again and again, for the life you're creating. Because the truth is, healing isn't the end of the road—it's the beginning of something bigger. And when you commit to this process, when you take responsibility for your body, your mind, and your future, you stop being just a survivor. You become the architect of a life you actually *want* to live.

In closing, I want to say something to those watching someone they care about go through this process. When you see them standing outside, searching for the right key to open the door, I know you want to run to them, unlock it yourself, and shout, "Look, it's open!" But the thing is, you can't. You can't open the door for them—but you *can* make sure they have the keys. You can gently place them in their hands, help them understand what each one does, and remind them that even when they feel lost, they're not alone. You can stand beside them as they fumble, as they hesitate, as they try the wrong key over and over again. And you can certainly make sure the deadbolt isn't locked—that there's nothing standing in their way except their own courage to step through. Because as much as you might want to throw the door wide open and pull them inside, healing is something they have to choose for themselves. You can't force them to walk through that doorway. But you *can* make sure that when they do—when they finally turn the key that fits, when the lock clicks open and the door swings wide—there's warmth waiting on the other side. You can create a space that feels safe, where they don't have to explain themselves, where they can simply *be.* You can remind them that they don't have to brace for impact anymore, that they don't have to stand in the doorway, unsure if they belong.

Because when they finally step inside, when they look around and realize this is real—that they *made it,* that they are *here*—you get to be the one who smiles and says, "Welcome home."

CHAPTER 13
HOPE

As we bring this book to a close, I want to tell you a little story about a tree—the red cedar. In the wild, this tree stands strong, its deep red heartwood rich with natural oils that repel rot and decay. Fungi, the silent invaders of the forest, should spell doom for this tree—breaking it down from the inside out. But the red cedar has a secret. The very thing meant to harm it—a toxic extract within its own bark—doesn't just defend against destruction, it triggers something remarkable. When exposed to small doses of this toxin, fungi that should have withered don't just survive—they grow stronger. They adapt. They thrive. This concept has a name: *hormesis*—the idea that a little bit of stress, a little bit of struggle, doesn't weaken, it fortifies. It sharpens. It prepares. At the cellular level, this process activates multiple genes that equip the organism to survive. It's not just poetic—it's biological.

The same principle has been seen in humans. Low levels of stress can trigger growth factors in the brain, strengthen the immune system, fuel energy metabolism, and even switch off harmful genes embedded in our DNA. The right kind of challenge doesn't just test us—it changes us. It builds us. And maybe that's the real legacy of healing. Not becoming someone new but returning to something ancient inside us—our inborn ability to adapt, endure, and emerge from the fire stronger than we were before.

I didn't ingest extracts from a red cedar tree, but I know what it means to be exposed to something that should have destroyed me. Trauma was my toxin. The long, relentless exposure to it should have rotted me from the inside out. Growing up with a father battling severe PTSD/PTSI symptoms, nearly losing my life to a boat propeller, watching my mother slip away in a tragic, unnecessary death—these were my fungi, creeping through my foundation, threatening to break me apart.

But something else happened: Instead of being consumed, I adapted. I grew. I became something different—something stronger than I ever imagined. Not because I was immune to suffering, but because I learned how to turn it into something useful. Resilience isn't built in comfort. It's carved out of struggle. And now, that very ability to withstand, to persevere, to push forward—it's what allows me to help others do the same. Here's what I want you to take from this: it's not the absence of adversity that makes us strong—it's learning how to face it, how to build tolerance to life's stressors, how to turn struggle into fuel. If you protect yourself from every hardship, if you shield yourself from every discomfort, you don't build resilience—you build fragility.

Because just like the red cedar—and, apparently, Kelly Clarkson—what doesn't kill you doesn't just make you stronger, it makes you unstoppable. Most people avoid stress like it's some kind of poison—dodging anything that might make them uncomfortable, from public speaking to difficult conversations, from new challenges to the unknown. But here's the truth: you can handle so much more than you think. Your body, your mind, your very biology is designed for survival—and not just survival: adaptation. What if, instead of fearing stress, you started using it to your advantage?

Reading through this book, you've seen example after example of people who have faced hardship and emerged stronger—not by avoiding struggle, but by stepping into it. Resilience isn't something you either have or you don't, it's something you build. And just like a muscle, the more you train it, the stronger it gets. So how do you build resilience? How do you turn stress into fuel instead of letting it consume you? When I think about what's helped me most—what keeps me grounded, moving forward, and growing—it comes down to four things. I call it **HERE: Humor, Exercise, Respect,** and **Exploration.** It's simple, but powerful.

H—Humor: The Ultimate Survival Tool

Laughter isn't just about lightening the mood—it's a biological hack for resilience. It's how we trick our brains into feeling safe, even when the world feels anything but. Humor helps reframe challenges, diffuse stress, and keep us connected to others, even in the hardest times. And if there's one thing I've learned, it's that the ability to laugh—especially at yourself—is a lifeline when life gets hard.

People are often surprised by my sense of humor. I think they expect me to be more serious, given my work, my research, and the topics I deal with every day. But if you spend enough time with me, you'll quickly realize that I crack a lot of jokes. I can't help it—it's just how I'm wired. My wife, however? *Not* as impressed. She's heard them all before, and let's just say, her tolerance is significantly lower than that of my patients and colleagues. I'd like to think that deep down, she appreciates my comedic genius. But the science is clear: laughter changes the brain. Studies show that humor actually impacts the amygdala—the part of the brain responsible for processing fear and stress—helping to regulate emotional responses. Brain scans have demonstrated that laughter increases connectivity between different regions of the brain, improving cognitive flexibility and emotional regulation. In other words, humor isn't just a distraction—it's a reset button for the nervous system.

Not all humor is created equal, though. Research suggests that positive, lighthearted humor boosts resilience, while gallows humor—the kind that leans too hard into cynicism—can actually make things worse. There's a fine line between using humor to cope and using it to avoid. The goal isn't to numb pain with jokes, but to use laughter as a way to stay connected to life, even in the darkest moments. Some of the most resilient people I've ever met—patients, soldiers, trauma survivors—have an incredible ability to find humor in the absurdity of life. It's not that they take their pain lightly; it's that they refuse to let it consume them. They laugh, not because life is easy, but because they know that sometimes, *laughter is the only thing that keeps you going.*

So, if you ever find yourself drowning in stress, try this: Watch a comedy special. Call the funniest person you know. Tell a bad joke. Even if it feels forced, even if it starts as nothing more than an exhale through your nose, give yourself permission to laugh. Your brain—and your future self—will thank you.

E—Exercise: The Medicine You Can't Afford to Skip

If I could put one thing at the top of the list for rewiring the brain after psychological trauma, it's movement. Exercise isn't just about looking good or getting stronger—it's about repairing the damage stress and trauma leave behind. It produces endorphins, the body's natural opioids, helping you feel calmer and more in control. It reduces inflammation, which is linked to anxiety, depression, and cognitive decline. It increases brain volume, particularly in the prefrontal cortex (where critical thinking happens) and the hippocampus (where memories are stored). These are two areas hit hardest by chronic stress and trauma, and exercise literally rebuilds them. It restores balance to the nervous system, helping shift from survival mode into a state where true healing can happen.

And you don't need to be an elite athlete to benefit. Any movement counts—walking, lifting weights, stretching, even dancing in your kitchen. The key is consistency. Every time you move, you're sending a message to your body: *we are safe, we are strong, we are capable.*

R—Respect: For Yourself and Your Limits

Respect isn't about pushing yourself to the breaking point—it's about knowing when to push and when to pause. It's about understanding that true strength isn't reckless endurance; it's *intentional* endurance. It's choosing when to step forward, when to stand firm, and when to step back—not out of weakness, but out of wisdom.

I used to think that stress had to be tackled head-on, that the only way to prove my strength was to grit my teeth and plow through. But that mindset is a trap: it leads to burnout, exhaustion, and a hollow version of resilience that looks strong on the outside but is crumbling underneath. Real resilience means respecting yourself enough to set boundaries. It means recognizing that your energy is a resource, not an unlimited supply, and that pushing yourself past your limits isn't heroism—it's self-sabotage.

One of the best pieces of advice I ever got was this: control what you can before stepping into what you can't. Before quitting my job at Rush University—a difficult, emotional decision—I didn't just throw myself into the stress of it. I took myself out for an incredible French dinner, had a glass of wine, let myself *fully relax*. Then, I faced what needed to be done. That moment sticks with me because it was a turning point in how I saw resilience. It wasn't about suffering through the moment—it was about preparing myself to handle it in the best way possible.

That's the difference between reckless endurance and *strategic* endurance. Reckless endurance says: Just push harder. Keep going. Ignore the warning signs. Strategic endurance says: Prepare yourself. Support yourself. Then, when it's time, step in fully.

Respecting yourself means knowing when to challenge yourself and when to give yourself grace. It means recognizing that rest is not the opposite of resilience—it's a crucial part of it. If you never slow down, never pause to refuel, never acknowledge your own needs, you're not strong—you're running on fumes. And that doesn't lead to success, it leads to collapse.

Think about it like this: if you had to cross a brutal, unforgiving landscape—a desert, a frozen tundra, a mountain range—you wouldn't just charge forward without preparation. You'd take time to gather supplies, plan your route, make sure you had food, water, and shelter. Your life is no different. The challenges you face require *you* to be strong, and that strength comes from respecting what you need to maintain it. So, before you push through another stressful situation, ask yourself: Have I taken care of myself first? Am I pushing forward because I'm ready, or because I think I *have* to? Is this stress necessary, or am I making things harder than they need to be? What can I control in this situation to make it easier on myself?

Resilience isn't about suffering for the sake of suffering. It's about showing up as your best self, and sometimes, that means treating yourself with care. It means choosing to prepare rather than endure, to rest rather than run on empty, to respect your limits rather than ignore them. Because resilience isn't about how much you can take—it's about how well you *recover.*

E—Exploration: The Cure for Stagnation

Curiosity has been a driving force in my life for as long as I can remember. I've always wanted to understand things—to pull them apart, look beneath the surface, figure out *why* something works the way it does. That curiosity has taken me down some strange and unexpected paths, and looking back, I can see how much it has shaped my resilience. Because at its core, resilience is about adaptability, and adaptability is fueled by curiosity. If you want to build resilience, you have to be willing to step into the unknown. You have to ask the questions no one else is asking. You have to look at your life—the parts that feel stagnant, unfulfilling, or just plain miserable—and get curious about what else is possible. If you're in a dead-end job, start looking at what else is out there, even if the thought of leaving terrifies you. If you're in a toxic relationship, recognize that the stress of staying is just as damaging as one big traumatic event. If you feel stuck in life, take a risk—travel somewhere new, start a hobby, meet new people. Change is uncomfortable because it's supposed to be. The brain doesn't like uncertainty. It clings to what it knows, even if what it knows is painful. But comfort zones don't build resilience—challenges do. And the mental turmoil that comes with change doesn't last forever. The effects of staying stuck, however, will.

I've seen this pattern play out in so many people—patients, friends, even in myself. We avoid change because we assume we're not ready. That we need to wait until we feel *sure*. But certainty never comes before action. *Curiosity* is what gets you moving. What if you asked yourself, *What else could this be*, instead of, *This is just how things are*? What if you saw your discomfort not as a warning sign, but as an invitation? What if you treated fear as a signal—not to stop, but to lean in? Because that's where real transformation happens: not in the places where everything is familiar and predictable, but in the moments where you push yourself to see what's on the other side of fear. Resilience isn't about "bouncing back" to who you were before trauma—it's about becoming something even stronger. Think about the red cedar tree. It doesn't resist stress—it *adapts.* It *transforms.* It *uses* stress to become more resilient, more durable, more unshakable.

The same thing happens in humans. Trauma and stress can rewire the brain in ways that accelerate aging, disrupt the immune system, and trigger chronic disease. But—and this is the part no one talks about—healing can rewire it back. Science shows that treating trauma can actually reverse the speed of aging and restore proper brain function. Mindfulness, therapy, movement, exploration—these aren't just "nice" things to do. They physically rebuild the brain, strengthening the connections that regulate stress, memory, and decision-making.

And the best part? You control the process. Exploration is a mindset. A refusal to settle. A willingness to see what else is possible. It's about standing at the edge of what's known, looking out at the vast, uncertain landscape ahead, and deciding to take a step forward anyway. Because growth isn't about avoiding stress—it's about proving to yourself that you can handle it.

So, take the risk. Face the challenge. Ask the hard questions. Let curiosity lead you to the life you haven't even imagined yet. Because the more you train yourself to step into the unknown, the stronger you become. And once you do? Nothing will ever hold you back again.

Hope: The Bridge Between Survival and Thriving

Resilience teaches you how to withstand. How to adapt. How to turn pain into fuel and keep moving forward, no matter how hard life tries to break you. But there's one more element—one that determines whether all this effort leads to a life of merely enduring, or a life of *thriving*. That element is **hope.**

Without hope, resilience is just grit without direction. Without hope, all the work you put into healing—changing habits, rewiring your brain, rebuilding your body—becomes a battle without a victory. You can exercise, eat well, face your fears, and still be stuck if, deep down, you don't believe there's something better waiting on the other side. *Hope is the difference between survival and truly living.* It's what allows you to envision a future beyond the pain. It's what turns healing into more than just an endless struggle to "get better"—it turns it into an opening, a doorway, a chance to create something new. And yet, when you've been through trauma, hope can feel like the hardest thing to hold on to. What happens when hope fades? Well, hopelessness isn't just a feeling. It's a neurological shutdown. It narrows your focus, dulls your senses, convinces you that nothing will ever change. The weight of trauma—whether it comes from a single catastrophic event or years of accumulated stress—alters the way you see the world, *literally.* Your brain stops looking for solutions. It stops scanning for possibility. Instead, it prepares for more pain. More loss. More of the same.

This is why people lose themselves in cycles of self-destruction. Not because they don't want to heal, but because they can't see a reason to. When hope disappears, survival mode takes over, making even the smallest efforts feel pointless. Hope, however, is not something you passively wait for. It's something you build. Most people think of hope as an emotion—something that either appears or it doesn't. But the truth is, hope is an active process. It's a muscle you strengthen through action, a habit you develop by proving to yourself that life can, in fact, change.

Hope grows when you experience small wins. When you see evidence—real, tangible proof—that effort leads to progress. When you notice that after a few weeks of exercising, you feel lighter. When therapy shifts the way you think. When you realize that no, you haven't been triggered in weeks, and that the anger, the panic, the old survival responses aren't running your life anymore.

Hope expands when you surround yourself with people who believe in you. Sometimes, you need to borrow hope from others. Remember the story of Tom and Jen Satterly? If you don't believe in yourself yet, let someone else hold the belief for you: a friend, a therapist, a mentor. Someone who says, "You don't see it yet, but I do. And I'm not letting go until you see it too."

Hope solidifies when you take action, even when you don't feel like it. You don't have to be bursting with hope to start. You just have to move forward. When you act *as if* things will get better, your brain starts believing they can.

Here, I want to acknowledge something very important: healing isn't linear. There will be setbacks. But as they used to say at County Hospital, "The measure of a person isn't how they end up in the crap—it's how they step out of it."

There will be days when hope feels distant. There will be moments when old patterns reassert themselves. This doesn't mean you're failing—it means you're human. The brain's default is to return to familiar patterns, even when those patterns cause suffering. This is why lasting change requires patience and persistence. Each time you recognize an old pattern and choose a different response, you're strengthening the neural pathways of healing. Each time you stumble and then find your way back to your practice, you're building resilience. The courage to begin again—to pick yourself up after a setback, to recommit to your healing journey even when progress seems slow—this is perhaps the truest expression of hope. It's the quiet knowing that tomorrow can be different from today, that you are not defined by your worst moments or your deepest wounds. This is why commitment matters more than motivation. Motivation fades. But when you stay consistent—when you keep doing the things that support your healing, even on the days you don't see immediate results—you build something unshakable.

The other thing I love about hope is that it is contagious. When you carry it, you spread it. When you hold onto it, even in the darkest times, you create possibility not just for yourself, but for others. Think about the people in your life. Who is still standing outside the house, searching for their key? Who is pressing their face against the glass, convinced they'll never belong inside? You can't open the door for them. As much as you might want to throw it wide open, as much as you might long to pull them inside and show them the warmth waiting on the other side, they have to find their own key. That's the hardest part of watching someone you love struggle. You can't do it for them. You can't force them to heal, to choose the right door, to turn the key in the lock.

But you *can* make sure they have the keys. You can be the person who says, *"Here's what worked for me."* You can offer them tools, share resources, and be a steady presence when they want to give up. And maybe most importantly, you can make sure that when they *do* find the key—when they finally step through that door—there is warmth waiting on the other side. A space that feels safe. A place where they are seen. A place where they can finally exhale and realize: *I made it. I'm home.*

This is how healing ripples outward. It's how generational trauma ends. It's how entire communities shift. When one person heals, they create a path for others to follow. Your journey doesn't end with personal healing. As you continue to grow and integrate your experiences, something remarkable happens: your resilience begins to affect others. The science of collective resilience shows that healing is contagious. When you regulate your nervous system, you help coregulate others around you. When you demonstrate that recovery is possible, you become living proof for those still struggling. Your journey creates ripples that extend far beyond your own life. This is perhaps the most powerful aspect of hope—its ability to transcend the individual and transform communities. In a world where trauma is endemic, your personal healing becomes an act of massive change. Some of you reading these words may go on to become formal guides for others—therapists, coaches, healers. Others will simply live your transformed lives in ways that inspire those around you. Either way, your healing matters not just for you, but for all those your life touches.

There's so much more I could say about hope, but instead, I'll leave you with a story my father once told me—a parable that has kept me going through the worst times:

Two frogs fall into a jug of milk. The first frog panics. He sees no way out. "I guess it is time to die," he sighs. He stops struggling, stops fighting, and lets himself sink. And just like that, he drowns.

The second frog is terrified, too. He doesn't see an immediate escape either. But he refuses to give in. "I will fight until the last possible moment," he declares. He kicks and paddles, even as exhaustion sets in. He doesn't know what else to do, so he just keeps moving. Minutes pass. Then hours. The milk around him begins to thicken. He doesn't understand what's happening, but he keeps going. Eventually, he realizes the milk has turned to butter. And in that moment, he has something solid beneath him—something to push against. He takes one last mighty leap and jumps out of the jug, free.

This is the power of persistence. This is the power of hope.

Because hope isn't passive. It's not sitting back, waiting for a miracle—it's action. It's refusing to sink, even when every muscle in your body is screaming for you to stop. It's choosing to believe in the possibility of change—even when you can't see it yet. And here's the part people don't talk about: *you don't have to see progress for progress to be happening.* The second frog didn't know the milk was thickening beneath him. He had no proof that his effort was doing anything at all. He just kept kicking. And that was enough. Sometimes, all you can do is *keep moving.* Keep showing up. Keep putting one foot in front of the other. Even when you're exhausted. Even when it feels pointless. Even when you have no idea how or when things will shift. Because the truth is, change is always happening beneath the surface. Your effort is never wasted.

And maybe that's where you are right now—kicking, paddling, exhausted, unsure if anything you're doing is making a difference. But let me tell you something: you're thickening the milk. Every time you choose to keep going, every time you refuse to let despair take over, you are creating the conditions for something to shift. For an opening to appear. For a moment to arise when suddenly—you have something solid beneath you. So, keep kicking. Keep fighting. Keep holding on. Because hope isn't just what gets you through. It's what gets you out.

As you close these pages, I offer not an ending but an invitation. An invitation to carry these tools, these insights, these keys with you as you continue your journey. An invitation to trust the process, even when the path isn't clear. An invitation to believe in your capacity to heal, to grow, to flourish. The fact that you've read this far is evidence of your commitment to transformation. It's evidence of hope already at work within you. Remember: *your body is designed to heal.* Your brain is built for adaptation and growth. Your spirit naturally moves toward wholeness. All the tools and practices we've explored are simply ways of removing obstacles and creating conditions for your innate healing capacity to flourish. You already have everything you need. The master key—hope—has been within you all along. It's what led you to open this book, to try new approaches, to keep reaching for a different experience.

Now, let that same hope guide you forward. Let it illuminate the path ahead, even when that path winds through uncertain terrain. Let it remind you that you are not broken, but breaking open into something more spacious, more healthy, more alive than you've yet imagined. Your journey continues. And with hope as your compass, *healing isn't just possible—it's inevitable.* May you walk forward with courage, with compassion for yourself and others, and with the unshakable knowledge that no matter what you've endured, the capacity for renewal lives within you. This is not the end. It's a new beginning. And it starts right now, with hope.

You don't have to stay stuck in old patterns. You don't have to be defined by trauma. You have the power to reshape your brain, your habits, your entire life. And the more you train yourself to step into stress—not recklessly, but strategically—the stronger you become. So, take the risk. Face the challenge. Say yes to something that scares you. Because resilience isn't about avoiding struggle—it's about proving to yourself that you can handle it. And once you do? Nothing will ever hold you back again.

So, if there's one thing I want you to take away from this book, it's this: you are capable of more than you've ever imagined. You've been tested. You've been through things that could have broken you. And yet, you're still here. Reading this. Looking for answers. Reaching for something better. That means something.

This journey—healing, resilience, stepping fully into your life—isn't just about getting back to who you were before trauma. It's about becoming something even stronger. And you can do it. The door is open. The keys are in your hands. You don't have to stand outside anymore. So, keep kicking. And get ready to jump.

Welcome home.